THE HINDU
SECRETS
OF
VIRILITY
AND
REJUVENATION

THE SCIENCE OF RESTORING
SEXUAL VITALITY

BY

JOSEPH ANDREW MARCELLO

Based upon an original text by

EMIL RAUX

Special Contents

Copyrighted 2016

by

Joseph A. Marcello

Printed in the United States of America

First Edition

ISBN-13: 978-1532968372
ISBN-10: 153296837X

TABLE OF CONTENTS

I

IN PURSUIT OF POTENCY

Be fruitful. . .

Genesis 1:28

The dictionary defines 'virility' as". . . the quality of having strength, energy, and a strong sex drive; manliness."

While these terms might be interpreted as chauvinistic by the mindset of some, what individual with XY chromosomes wouldn't want to have strength, energy, and a strong sex drive in his tank?

Or, in the immortal words of Irving Mills', 'It don't mean a thing if it ain't got that swing. . .'

The quest for virility has been with us as long as humans have walked the earth, but it has largely been one oriented toward external solutions—in ancient times, arcane alchemical formulas involving rare plant and animal substances; at the turn of the 19th century, radical surgical procedures such as Voronoff's monkey gland transplants; and, in our own era, libido-enhancing pharmaceutical drugs—with side effects ranging from loss of vision and hearing to chest pain. It seems mankind has been willing to do just about anything to preserve its procreative prowess—whether the intent was reproduction or pleasure.

But all too often, such measures have proved to be short-lived and ineffective, leaving their adherents no better for their pains and expense.

1

Yet, throughout history, there have been individuals who have been able to defy the odds and retain their sexual vitality—even into their seventh, eighth, ninth decades and beyond.

A very recent example may suffice to silence any would-be skeptics:

"Randy Ramjit and his 52-year-old wife, Shakuntala Devi, gave birth to a healthy baby boy earlier this month.

The nonagenarian enjoys a healthy sex life with his partner who says the former wrestler 'can make love like any 25-year-old man.'

As a bachelor for almost nine decades, the pensioner credits his healthy diet as the secret to a long life—and abstinence from drugs and alcohol.

'I do it three or four times a night,' he told reporters outside his home in Haryana, India. 'My neighbours are jealous and they keep asking me for my secret, but all I tell them is that it is God's will.

'I'm healthy and I enjoy sex with my wife. I think it's very important for a husband and wife to have sex regularly, and when she asks I will go on all night, but for the sake of my child I've put our needs aside for now.

'I care for my wife and I give her everything she needs. She is a very happy woman.'

The pensioner hit the headlines in 2010 when he became the world's oldest father at 94, beating a previous record set by an Indian farmer Nanu Ram Jogi when he was 90 in 2007."

In further testimony of her husband's sexual prowess Shakuntala offers the following:

"'It doesn't matter how old he is, I love him and I care for him dearly even though he shouts at me sometimes. . .He doesn't seem old to me, he can make love like any 25-year-old man, even better because he can go on all night, and he makes a wonderful father."

(Source: The Daily Mail (UK)/ http://metro.co.uk)

Clearly, it would seem, it is possible for even men of very advanced age to retain potency—and in the lady's estimation—to perform passionately.

However, apart from such exceptional cases, and even in spite of the proliferation of contemporary medical knowledge, males in the 21st century are at greater risk of infertility—and even outright impotence--than ever before. Below are listed a few of the conclusions by Wolf-Bernhard Schill in his research paper, *Fertility and sexual life of men after their forties and in older age*:

Weakened generation of sperm
Disappearance of the circadian testosterone (T) rhythm.
Complete infertility in one third of men over 60.
Complete infertility in 50% of men over 80.
Reduced bioavailability of sex hormones.
Lower testosterone concentrations in men over 60.
Reduced virility
Reduced oxygen to testicles

Disappearance of the circadian rhythm
Decreased muscle mass
Decline in production of testosterone
Reduced strength
Reduced sexual hair growth
Lower libido
Erectile dysfunction
Age-related decline in androgen and plasma testosterone
Atrophy of seminiferous tubules
Decrease in the number of 700 million Leydig cells in a
20- year-old man by 6 to 7 million per year

In spite of this litany of pathological changes, Schill concludes, "In principle, however, spermatogenesis may be retained well into senescence. Children have been fathered by men over 90 years."

The very real possibility of lifelong potency is emphatically reaffirmed in the present republication of Emile Raux's *Hindu Secrets of Virility and Rejuvenation*, a long out-of-print, all-but-forgotten manual of ancient wisdom that harbors the potential to retain one's virility, or to restore it in the event that it has been lost. Raux distills into simple, easily-performed movements the essence of long-concealed Indian rejuvenation practices.

To his credit, Emile Raux was unequivocal in his conviction that the Hindu Secrets could do all that might ever be hoped of them, and goes so far as to assure his readers, *"In the next few pages you will be introduced to these age-old and ageless virility secrets of the Hindus. They do not apply alone to those who have let their virility slip away, but to those as well who wish to remain until the very end of their lives*

*free of the barren disillusionment of impotence, free of weakness
of all kinds; free men, whole men!"*

The Hindu dands — or exercises — are nothing more than four simple movements designed for the renewal of the nervous and glandular systems, and for their ability to empower our vital life-functions — especially the procreative. Raux did not concern himself with the psychological aspects of maintaining one's virility, which, while relevant, have no essential place in his manuscript. It is enough to know that, when we have renewed ourselves at the organic level, and there are no physical blockages or psychological resistances, we will have the life-force to express ourselves fully in any direction we choose — artistically, athletically or sexually, as the case may be.

Little wonder, then, that a culture that preceded the birth of Christ by some two millennia should have had ample time to gather deeper knowledge about the workings of the human system and how best to care for it.

In the almost three quarters of a century since the publication of the *Hindu Secrets*, much valuable additional information pertaining to the restoration of virility has come to light in traditional and contemporary health research, embracing such diverse fields as endocrinology, sexology, psychology, nutrition, Taoism and other esoteric and exoteric sources. The most important of these new findings has also been included to complement the basic practice of the Hindu Secrets.

Emil Raux's offering is as timely now as when it first appeared, and while it does not pretend to be an encyclopedic treatise on its subject, it provides a critically important missing piece in the acquisition and cultivation of sexual health.

There is ample reason to believe that the information contained in this volume, if faithfully implemented, has the potential to take its practitioners a very long way toward fulfilling that goal. While the Hindu Secrets are, in and of themselves, powerful tools for the restoration of potency, they will much more rapidly achieve their intended purpose if they are supported by a nutritional matrix that provides the raw materials necessary for glandular and neurological rejuvenation.

There are many substances from the natural world that have a marked effect upon enhancing our life energy in general as well as our sexual reserves in particular—yet this is not, even now, common knowledge. For this reason several chapters have been devoted to an in-depth exploration of various valuable botanicals.

For, once the Hindu Secrets begin to leverage their deep stimulation upon the system, there will be all the more need for nutrients, enzymes, minerals and other support factors the body requires.

Ideally, the Hindu Secrets should be faithfully practiced while the body is consistently supplied with a rich array of rejuvenative elements are being made available. This two-pronged approach would ensure that, once re-activated, the vital centers of the body would have ready access to the essential nutrients it requires.

Nor is Raux hung up on the purely sexual aspects of maintaining virility, compelling as these may be—he has the depth of insight to know that the aquifer of virility fuels not only a man's procreative life—but also his moral, spiritual and intellectual existence, all of which will founder and die without the underlying power conferred by optimal creative energy:

> ". . .as long as sex powers remain unimpaired, a man will feel dauntless, invincible, courageous, but once they wane he feels helpless. For everything a man does, his enjoyment of work, his power to achieve, his health, his courage, is dependent upon his sexual power. A strong, vital, normally-sexed body is one of the greatest assets a man may possess."

The etymology of the word 'holy' reveals it to be not so much a religious term as an existential one; as a direct descendant of the root-word 'halig,' meaning 'whole'; contrary to popular mythology, it denotes neither piety nor religiosity, but rather completeness, entirety, fulfillment of the natural design or destiny, whether of an oak tree, an elephant or a human being. To be holy, then, to be entire, full-fledged, lacking nothing—in other words, all that we were originally designed and destined to be.

While scholars and literary sleuths may continue to be intrigued by—and choose to pursue—the origin of the Hindu Secrets, such distractions need not delay those who truly wish to discover for themselves the validity of their effectiveness. Whether of Indian, Tibetan or some as yet unknown origin, the clear fact is that, through the centuries, far older, wiser cultures than ours have elected to practice and pass on the movements, bolstered by deep faith in their promised benefits, when performed as described:

II

HOW THE HINDU SECRETS WORK THEIR MAGIC

While the Hindu Secrets may at first seem like just so much arcane hocus pocus, upon close inspection they turn out to be a surprisingly scientific set of movements.

If we were to ask any knowledgeable physician or physiologist the single most essential component of life and well-being—or for that matter, healing and regeneration—the answer might well be: "Good circulation."

Unimpeded circulation—of lymph, blood and oxygen—is critical to life, health and optimal function. When circulation—no matter of which system--breaks down or totally ceases, so do the processes of life.

The major physiological difference between a healthy, functional person and an unhealthy, dysfunctional one is the viability of these three circulatory systems.

In the classic *Textbook of Medical Physiology by* Guyton and Hall—a must for all first year medical students—we learn that if the lymphatic system were to shut down for 24 hours, certain death would ensue, so critical is the waste disposal function for detoxification and maintaining a clean cell environment.

Likewise, if the bloodstream were obstructed for even a brief time, certain death would quickly follow, for it is the chief carrier for both tissue oxygen and nutrients.

And it hardly needs saying that a major obstruction in the respiratory system would immanent death within a matter of minutes or even seconds.

On the positive side, circulation is no less critical to the processes of healing and regeneration, whether these be of cells, tissues or organs. Without adequate blood flow, air flow and lymphatic drainage, there would be no possibility for repair and reconstruction, no matter how heroic the medical treatment.

The best diets, costliest supplements and most powerful pharmaceuticals in the world can do nothing without the round-the-clock nutrient-delivery and waste-removal that good circulation provides.

But with sufficient attention to maintaining the health of these three circulatory systems, it is possible to dramatically reduce the time required to cleanse, nourish and rebuild cells, tissues and organs that have experienced injury or enervation due to faulty lifestyle or prolonged stress.

An impressive demonstration of this principle comes from Dr. Harold Riley, author of *The Edgar Cayce Handbook of Health and Healing,* who was, for many years, the primary physical therapist for the Association for Research and Enlightenment in Virginia Beach, Virginia; he relates the case of a weight-lifter who was asked to lift a certain weight as many times as he could until muscle fatigue prevented his continuing any further—a total some 900 odd times. After an interval of several minutes' rest he was asked to repeat the task, whereupon he was only able to lift the weight 400 times. However, when the same experiment was repeated with Dr. Riley providing a brief period of therapeutic massage to the arms of the lifter, he was almost able to match his first total.

In another experiment, researchers biopsied and screened tissue samples from the massaged and unmassaged legs of test subjects to compare the rates of their respective repair processes, and find out what difference massage would make on them, as vigorous exercise causes tiny tears in muscle fibers, leading to an immune reaction—inflammation—as the body begins repairing the injured cells.

They found that massage reduced the production of compounds called cytokines, which play a critical role in inflammation. Massage also stimulated mitochondria, the tiny powerhouses inside cells that convert glucose into the energy essential for cell function and repair.

Dr. Mark A. Tarnopolsky, a professor of pediatrics and medicine at McMaster University in Hamilton, explained, "The bottom line is that there appears to be a suppression of pathways in inflammation and an increase in mitochondrial biogenesis," helping the muscle adapt to the demands of increased exercise. He added that massage works quite differently from non-steroidal and other anti-inflammatory drugs, which reduce inflammation and pain but may actually retard healing. "There's some theoretical concern that there is a maladaptive response in the long run if you're constantly suppressing inflammation with drugs. With massage, you can have your cake and eat it too—massage can suppress inflammation and actually enhance cell recovery."

What would have taken the body from several hours to perhaps even several days to accomplish was accomplished in a matter of mere minutes, due to the benefits of the massage drainage techniques. These experiments confirmed that, with enlightened intervention, it is entirely possible to up-regulate the body's rate of self-healing and rejuvenating.

Likewise, the benefits attendant upon faithful practice of the Hindu Secrets are a direct result of their intensive focus upon the cerebrospinal axis which, once cleared of obstructions and rendered flexible, provides a potent stimulus to each of the seven endocrine centers—the pituitary, pineal, thyroid, thymus, adrenals and gonads.

Practicing these movements for even a brief time seldom fails to yield very palpable results, as they powerfully stimulate the system to come to a state of heightened integrity. This upgrade is far more than merely muscular—or of improved joint and ligament flexibility; it is first and foremost an energetic effect that extends not only to the purely physical—but which impacts the neurological, mental and spiritual levels as well. One eventually comes to feel a deep reservoir of psychophysical power accruing, a vital energy upon which one can draw—for physical, sexual or spiritual objectives, as desired.

Doing them over an extended period of time opens the doors of perception to far deeper, more subtle levels of practice—making their performance increasingly more rewarding.

III

THE TIBETAN CONNECTION

Readers who have had an opportunity to read Peter Kelder's *The Eye of Revelation*—later popularized as *Ancient Secrets of the Fountain of Youth* and *The Five Tibetan Rites of Rejuvenation*—will readily recognize the uncanny similarity—even absolute identicality—of the last four of those exercises to the dands of the present volume.

In-depth research by antiquarian bookman Jerry Watt has revealed that the first publication of *The Hindu Secrets of Virility and Rejuvenation* preceded the original appearance of *The Eye of Revelation* by just under a year, marking it as the true progenitor of these much-loved rejuvenation practices.

The order of exercises differs in the two approaches, and *The Eye of Revelation* included an additional spinning movement, classifying it as the first Rite of the five.

Watt is quite certain that the similarity of *The Eye of Revelation* to *The Hindu Secrets* is no accident, but rather the result of a strategic purloining of Raux's work by one Harry J. Gardener, an eccentric literary opportunist who authored dozens of books on self-development during the early-mid 20th century.

It is also noteworthy that, apart from this singular upright spinning movement—one in which there is virtually no flexure of the spine to speak of, the other rites or dands are essentially horizontal in nature, and rely for their respective rejuvenative effect upon a fairly intensive flexing of the spinal column.

Whatever the origin of the dands or rites may ultimately be discovered to be, it is interesting to note that the follow-up volume to *Ancient Secrets of the Fountain of Youth*, *Ancient Secrets of the Fountain of Youth Book II* shares many accounts of contemporary practitioners who have reaped a host of impressive benefits from their practice of these exercises—from heightened energy to recovery from serious and longstanding illness.

The critical message here is that one need not be led astray in a long and possibly futile quest for validation if the goods in hand prove worthy in practice.

This book is not intended, then, so much for scholars or researchers, but for those who are interested in preserving or restoring their life-energy and sexual vitality; if practiced faithfully, there is abundant evidence demonstrating that fruits will be forthcoming.

Raux's original manuscript steers clear of any sensationalism or excess and yet it offers, in its gentlemanly and pragmatic way, untapped treasures for those in the new millennium. While these dynamic practices closely resemble several of those from the yoga tradition, they do not strictly constitute yoga as such—but nor are they merely calisthenic movements. They are, instead, a clear, extraordinarily well-designed series of range-of-motion exercises that, when undertaken as prescribed, provide the body the opportunity for a physiological 'reset.'

With regard to those of the female gender who wish to practice the dands but who may feel marginalized by the exclusively male orientation of the text, there need be no conflict or concern. The cerebrospinal stimulation that the dands provide will prove equally beneficial to the female reproductive and endocrine centers as to the male.

In the final analysis, there is only one sure way to know whether or not Emile Raux's far-reaching claims are valid—and that is to faithfully perform the dands yourself—then judge whether or not a major transformation in your health and sexual vitality are under way.

If our experience is any guide, your efforts will not be in vain.

IV

THE POWER OF AWARENESS

Awareness is power. In our media-dominated culture, double-tasking is nearing epidemic proportions—having lunch working at their computer, or supper while to the TV. While our bodies may be engaged in the process of eating, the percentage of our attention that is actively experiencing their food—the scents, flavors, colors and textures—is marginal at best, and largely co-opted by the virtual world. When such a minimal fraction of our energy is actually present for an experience, we have almost no sense of ever having actually had it. We have "missed the moment"—and, in this case, the meal—because we were— no pun intended—"out to lunch," and failed to show up for the occasion, with the inner sense that it never quite really happened.

In a classic experiment, one group of women was served soup and given large spoons while a second group was given small spoons. At the end of the meal the women who had eaten with the small spoons reported uniformly greater satiety, with many of them unable to finish the entire bowl, while those with large spoons who ate more quickly were less satisfied.

But if we give full, expansive attention to our food, savoring each mouthful until it dissolves into our system, we have a far deeper experience that fills our entire sensorium, from eyes to nose to mouth stomach and beyond, with a feeling of having been truly nourished. After taking our nourishment in this way, there is no further desire for fulfillment.

Is it any wonder, then, that so many people find themselves addicted to nonstop consumption, and that relatively few seem to go through life with a sense of physical satisfaction?

Active, undivided attention is a potent facilitator in the success of every undertaking. The coordination of body and mind succeeds because the performance of the outer activity has an underlying energetic infrastructure to support it.

The same is true of the Hindu Secrets: once we release all distractions and devote ourselves—mind, feelings and body—to the dands, we will discover layer upon layer of unsuspected benefits and insights.

Whoever perseveres will experience deep benefits from the deceptively simple dands, and their aftereffects will linger long within one's physical and spiritual being.

I have taken the liberty of adding a brief final section on several highly effective lifestyle adjuncts which, while not strictly part of the Hindu Secrets, strongly support the seminal practices laid out in this book.

Here, then, for the first time, after an absence of three-quarters of a century, is the original text, complete with the author's accompanying photographs, of Emile Raux's *The Hindu Secrets of Virility and Rejuvenation.*

V

THE HINDU SECRETS OF VIRILITY AND REJUVENATION

(Original Text & Photographs)

༈༈༈

FOREWORD...

THE MOST important thing in any man's life is his virility. It is the touchstone to his success, to his happiness, to his health, to his long life. Without it, his life is barren; with it, his life is full, is real, is joyous. It follows. therefore, that to live a complete and a successful life, a man must have virility. If he has had the misfortune to lose his, he must regain it; if he still has virility, he must do something to keep it, so that it may last as long as life.

What is virility? In its broadest sense virility is the sum total of all the qualities which make a man a man— masculinity, forcefulness, procreative ability, vigor, aliveness. Virility is a quality which radiates from those who have it. It is much more than brute force or athletic prowess. It is health.

It is alertness. It is enthusiasm. It is tolerance. It is endurance. In short virility is the prime quality of manhood—and a man is not a whole man without it.

In this course you will learn age—old secrets of virility from an ancient and a very profound and learned race of men—the Hindu sages of India.

THE HINDU SECRETS OF VIRILITY AND REJUVENATION
THE ART OF RESTORING SEXUAL VITALITY

Long before the Christian era, long before the dawn of present-day medical science, these scholars had discovered secrets which we today are only beginning to perceive— secrets of how any man, if he choose, can retain his vigor and virility and manhood; secrets of how men who, through misfortune or neglect, have lost these precious qualities can regain them and be complete men once more.

As you read this course and begin putting into practice its precepts remember this: These methods are tested and proved by the ages. For two thousand years they have been in use. ·

Millions of men have benefited by them.

You also will benefit.

Virility in Everyday Life

PSYCHIATRISTS and doctors are coming more and more to realize that one of the chief causes of human unhappiness and failure is failing virility. They are also discovering that by restoring a man his virility they can make him happy and useful once more.

There is nothing more humiliating to a man than the feeling that he is no longer virile. Life for such a man holds nothing. He is degraded in his own eyes. He lives without a single illusion, his whole existence a barren plain. You do not expect greatness in such a man. You do not expect even ordinary success. For he is capable of neither.

But watch the change when this man is transformed into a virile, sturdy, intrepid, forceful male through the restoration of these vital processes!

Life then holds everything. The man is happy again.

He can overcome the depressing and discouraging situations of life which formerly made existence a peril and a trial.

The fact is that a man is only strong when he is strong inside and out—and that is the condition which we describe is normal virility--- the condition it is the purpose of this course to teach you how to restore or retain.

THE HINDU SECRETS OF VIRILITY AND REJUVENATION
THE ART OF RESTORING SEXUAL VITALITY

Quite naturally the basis of all virility is the procreative instinct and ability of man. Another name for it is sex. From the moment of conception, throughout our life to its very end, we are controlled by this force of sex. So we may say that sex is the most important part of our existence. And as long as sex powers remain unimpaired, a man will feel dauntless, invincible, courageous, but once they wane he feels helpless. For everything a man does, his enjoyment of work, his power to achieve, his health, his courage, is dependent upon his sexual power. A strong, vital, normally-sexed body is one of the greatest assets a man may possess.

Virility is the gift of every man, but, unfortunately, because of the pace of our modern lives and the unnatural conditions with which we are surrounded and the abuses to which we subject ourselves, too many men lose this priceless gift.

Nature never intended that man's sex powers should wither and wane. Mark this: there is every evidence that these powers should last as long as life.

In a normal man they do.

To the Hindus, for example, it is unthinkable that a man should ever be less than a complete man.

They regard impotence as a sin, weakness as an admission of ignorance in the art of preserving and caring for the most sacred heritage of life.

When the late Lincoln Steffens, American reformer and author, married late in life and became, at the age of 60, the father of a son, much was made over the fact. He was pointed out as an example of extreme virility; a man to look at with envious eyes. In India, he wouldn't have got passing notice. Among the intelligent Hindus, fatherhood at 60, 70, 80, 90 is accepted as the normal thing, as it should be here, because the retention of the vital powers is neither difficult nor mysterious. It is normal.

And yet when Dr. Gilbert Van Tassel Hamilton, noted American physician, made his careful study of American men to determine their degree of virility, he found that 45 out of one hundred admitted they were sub-normal in virility and actually, to some degree, impotent!

Do you wonder when you read things like this that there is so much unhappiness, so much failure, so much discouragement?

For hundreds of years men have sought some magic by which to restore their youth and their virility, by which to overcome the condition which is so oppressive when it comes. Most of their quests have been ludicrous if not pitiful. You remember the search for the fountain of youth. . .the nostrums of many kinds . . . more recently the expensive and dangerous surgical operations . . . the electric treatments . . . the incantations. All these and many others have been invoked in the fruitless quest for virility by men who realize that virility is the all in all of life.

And all during the time they sought, within them was the secret of restoration which would have made them whole again and new, if they could but have perceived the secret and put it to use.

In the next few pages you will be introduced to these age-old and ageless virility secrets of the Hindus. They do not apply alone to those who have let their virility slip away, but to those as well who wish to remain until the very end of their lives free of the barren disillusionment of impotence, free of weakness of all kinds; free men, whole men!

The next chapter introduces you to these priceless secrets of the Hindus, shows you how they were discovered and what they have meant to scores of generations of mankind.

The Hindus Discover the Secret

ALMOST from the beginning of time there has been a search for secrets virility and rejuvenation. Men have never doubted that somewhere these secrets could be found. Indeed, in the Bible itself you are assured that "man shall renew his youth like an eagle," and that. "thou shalt be as in the morning. having rebuilded thy body in the night."

The greatest scholar of the Middle Ages, Roger Bacon, wrote in his tremendous book, The Opus Majus, that: "God the most High and Glorious has prepared a means of preserving health and for combating the ills of old age and retarding them," and a modern scholar, Dr. Robert Bell Burke of the University of Pennsylvania, assures us that: "There truly was a medicine which was successfully used to prolong youth and life."

Aristotle, the Greek sage and philosopher, wisest of the ancients, centuries before Bacon lived alluded to "a medicine called the ineffable glory and treasure of the philosophers, which completely rectifies the whole human body."

The one fundamental error which these scholars all made was that of searching for what they termed a "medicine" from the outside. The Hindus were wiser. They looked for it where they knew they would find it: inside the man, not from an outside source. And no one else has ever discovered it but these Hindu sages. What you will learn in this course are the secrets for which men for centuries sought in vain.

That the Hindus should discover the secrets of virility and rejuvenation is natural enough. No other race has ever developed the profound philosophical thought of these sages of the East. Nor has any other nation so completely deified sex and sexual relations and sexual power. Upon the adoration of procreative and sexual Shakti (power) seen throughout nature, hinges the Hindu faith. Hindus worship generative power. So do we. But we have a sense of modesty which makes us hide our worship in shame; whereas, in India they sanctify sexual love to a greater degree than elsewhere in the world.

Whenever any people will make so important an issue of any subject or theme or idea, they will become masters of it—and know far more about it than will those who treat it casually or secretly or with apologies. For centuries the great Hindu books on sex and the art of love have vaguely hinted that behind this art was some secret of rejuvenation never revealed to outside eyes. You read allusions to it in the Kama Sutra, perhaps the greatest of all Hindu books on the art of love; in the *Anango Rango*, the *Panca Sayaka*, the *Smara Dipika*, the *Kali Shastra* and others.

But so carefully has the actual secret been guarded that it is doubtful if more than a handful of Americans know what it is.

You see, the whole Hindu philosophy of rejuvenation and the rebuilding and retention of virility rests upon the belief that these vital energies must be conserved where

25

they belong and virility piled up within the body into the organs and glands and tissues by a simple process of continual stimulation, rather than permitted to become dissipated and wasted.

This is a commonsense approach to an important subject, you will agree.

Hindus do not believe that surgical operations help or should ever be practiced. They are unnecessary. They are dangerous. Medicines they hold to be worse than useless. Mechanical means of rejuvenation are a folly. All that is necessary is that man should learn how to conserve and develop these forces of his, and they will last as long as long as he does.

No man knows when the Hindus first discovered their secrets. We do know, from their ancient writings, that as long ago as 2,000 years the secrets were known and the methods were being employed in practically the same form as are in use to this day.

Originally these methods started as religious rites, sacred activities that were part of the profound faith of the Hindus of those ancient times. Soon it was discovered that they had a value entirely apart from their spiritual worth: they stimulated the body and its glands, they rejuvenated them, they "renewed his youth like an eagle" of the man who practiced them. So they gradually evolved into a philosophical and a physical system for the benefit of the centuries.

They are a secretive race, these Hindus, and when the Europeans conquered their country they did not rush out and blatantly advertise their secrets. Indeed, it was generations before western scholars began to have an inkling of this fascinating art of rejuvenation and, many scholars even to this day know next to nothing about it, just as they know nothing or next to nothing about most of the institutions which give India its inscrutable aura of mystery.

As a matter of fact, these secrets are not the possession of every one in India by any means. To the low caste masses they are as much unknown as to the rank and file of our own country. It is only among the high caste Hindus, the students of nature and life, the scholars, the philosophers, that this method of rejuvenation is known and practiced.

But among them its efficacy is beyond any doubt one of the marvels of the East. Used these methods have produced physical specimens of manhood such as no other nation of the world has ever seen. By following the simple methods you will presently be taught, a race of supermen developed itself. Europe first saw them in 1908, these mighty men from India, when they came as a troupe to London to engage in physical combat with the best athletes of England and France. The contests were travesties, so superior were the East Indians. They overcame the best athletes of Europe in few seconds' time.

And these men seem to retain their athletic and virile power, throughout life. They remain full men in every sense of the word, though they live, as many do, to the ages of 85, 90 and even older. Their powers do not wane. Their masculine vigor does not abate.

The price they pay for virility is a small price indeed. There is nothing complicated about the system which develops them. There is nothing strenuous about it. They do not submit to painful operations, take rest cures or dope themselves with pills. They follow a few minutes of simple daily routine.

That is all.

But behind their daily practices lie 2,000 years of studious application by scholars to discover the true secrets of virility. So they use, as part of their daily life, a great conservation and development and rejuvenating force—the secret of their race.

It is this same system which you will be taught a little later on by this course. It is this same system which, when it becomes a part of your daily life, will enable you to reach some of your fondest desires in becoming and remaining more virile, more vigorous.

The Seat of Virility

To UNDERSTAND the basis of the Hindu Secrets and to see their practical application to your own daily life, you must read this brief chapter on the anatomy of the procreative or sex or vital organs of man.

The cradle of virility development is the pelvis—a basin-like structure which forms a bony girdle joining the lower limbs to the body and consisting of two hip bones and the sacrum.

The sacrum is a composite bone formed by the union of the vertebrae between the lumbar and the caudal regions. In this pelvic girdle repose all the sex organisms and forces. The pelvic girdle in reality is the cradle of virility.

Here are the organs and the glands which contribute sex sources to form the spermatozoa that creates life. Here repose the energies that first begin to wane within the body and bring about the aging of physical structure. Here also repose the forces which, properly stimulated by Hindu methods, can be rejuvenated so that the body springs into new life.

The pelvis has both a front and a back. The front of the pelvis is the abdominal wall. In Hindu rejuvenation it plays an important role. The procreative sources are

29

deeply seated within the pelvic girdle, but they are definitely affected by an unnatural looseness or sagging of the abdomen. If it is allowed to hang loosely and sag, the procreative sources which it protects cannot maintain vigor and tone and health. They deteriorate. Impotency is not far beyond the time when degenerative sagging of the abdomen sets in.

Keep in mind the abdominal phase of the pelvic girdle. It will be important a little later when you learn the Hindu Secrets.

The back of the pelvic region is the spine, which is held in place by a series of muscles. The most important of these are the erector spinal muscles, which form on each side of the spine from one end to the other.

The region of the spine at the pelvis is called the lumbar region. It is the body's hinge. Every day a thousand movements take place at this hinge. You twist; the hinge moves. You bend over; the hinge is moved. You lean backward; the hinge knows it. Every movement of the body puts work on the hinge.

Each of these movements destroys a modicum of muscle tissue; action, however slight, always does. Fatigue toxin accumulates wherever muscular tissue is destroyed. In time this fatigue toxin, unless carried away, pollutes and clogs the region with debris. The result of this is lowered vitality.

This disintegration is a perfectly normal, perfectly natural matter. The trouble is that at the hinge of the body the waste matter is seldom carried away as completely as it ought to be. So there is a slight secretion between the cartilaginous pads of the vertebrae. As a result this area of the body becomes stagnant, weak, and less effective. And you suffer from what you call pains "in the small of the back" or you feel a weakness there.

Perhaps you never knew before why weakness makes itself felt first at this vital region. It's because it is the most used, the hardest worked portion of the body. And it is also one of the most important parts, because it is the very heart of the vital regions.

Now, unless the front and the back protective walls of the pelvic girdle are maintained, virility is not possible. In the ordinary man they are not only not maintained: they are abused. Do you wonder at the high degree of sexual weakness and impotency that exists?

And then come the glands, the most important organs in the body in maintaining virility, because virility is a matter of glands.

Modern science has of late years proved what those ancient Hindus knew from antiquity: that the completely rejuvenated human body lies in the endocrine glands.

Because of the importance of glands in this virility-building process you should know something about them and what they do. It isn't necessary to become technical nor scientific to give you this picture.

The sex glands or glands of reproduction are called the gonads. They are closely interlocked with every other function of the human body. The ductless glands of the body, aside from the seminal vesicles, are these: the prostate, Cowper's, adrenal, thyroid, thymus and pituitary.

Now read a swift description of each and its function:

The seminal vesicles are two in number. They are pouches lying in back of the bladder, in front of the rectum. They serve as reservoirs for the semen.

The prostate, composed of glandular tissues, surrounds the neck of the bladder. Normally firm but not hard, it's about the size of a chestnut. At the moment of ejaculation the prostate ejects a milky fluid into the semen. The seat of much trouble is this prostate gland. Indeed, its condition is taken as a pretty good indication of the sexual health of a man.

Cowper's glands are tiny. Each is the size of a pea. There are two of them. Their place is just below the prostate. They also contribute to the seminal discharge.

Next come the adrenals—one resting on each kidney. They have a tendency to hold the gonads somewhat in check; yet if they are below par the testicles cannot function. The adrenals are normally stimulated and made to function the next gland we will consider: the thyroid.

This is not in the pelvic region at all, but in the neck, just above the collar bones. But it is closely related with every action that takes place in the f pelvic nevertheless, for it stimulates the adrenals and the gonads as well. If the thyroid is abnormal it affects the next gland on our list— the pituitary.

Another very small gland is this (it's about the size of a pea like the Cowper's). Its situation is within the head at the base of the brain about midway from front to back. Its condition has a marked influence on the condition of the gonads. Let it be subnormal and they fail to function. Let it be removed and impotence is inevitable.

There is one more. It is the thymus. Called "the gland of youth," the thymus, which is found just below the thyroid, is most active in puberty, when it has an important function in holding in check the sexual development of the child. Gradually it withers—but if this happens too suddenly old age comes on prematurely.

Even from this tabloid picture of the glands (which are really so complex that no one has ever understood them thoroughly) one thing has struck you: the close interconnection among them. One depends upon the other. Each assists the others to function properly. If one is deranged the system is thrown out of gear and ill results follow quickly.

Although our knowledge of glands is of comparatively recent origin, in some way the Hindu ··sages understood the function of these mysterious bodies and in their own way, without the benefit of modern medical science and research, devised means if to keep them normally stimulated and normally functioning.

When you learn the Hindu system of virility-building please notice that there is a method of stimulating each of these important glands, even, indeed, to the tiny pituitary; a simple, natural way of bringing gentle stimulation to keep each one functioning normally and properly throughout life.

Unless the pelvic girdle is kept in proper condition, both front and back; unless every one of the glands is stimulated, not harshly and unnaturally, but gently, continually, virility will vanish as inevitably as night follows day.

It is only by toning up these vital regions, only by giving them daily stimulation that a man can hope to remain a complete man all his days.

This truth the Hindus saw two thousand years ago.

This truth, when you put it into practice today, will help keep you virile, active, in the full health of mind, and body, and vital powers.

But unless something is done to preserve this normal balance among the procreative sources and the glands, impotence will come sooner or later—once a man suffers from the degradation of experiencing that, he will tell you that no other tragedy can so destroy a man's self-confidence, self-respect and joy of living. And yet impotence is one of the commoner conditions of modem life.

IMPOTENCE AND ITS RELIEF

A few pages back you learned that impotence, one of life's more bitter tragedies, is also one of modern life's more common tragedies—with 45 men out of 100 actually suffering blight and the other 55 not knowing when the awful truth will burst in upon them.

Scarcely another affliction can be imagined that is worse than the feeling of being impotent. It humiliates a man with all his being, leaves him completely disillusioned and bitter, leaves him without a single moment of mercy. Always he faces the fact that he who was once a man is no longer a man, but a half-man, an incomplete male being. But every man faces that future—unless he does something to circumvent it.

The insidious thing about impotence is the suddenness with which it often strikes. Without warning it comes. He who was a whole man yesterday, is incapable of being called a man today. Of course, the condition which brought impotence on did not start so suddenly: it was in the making for months, perhaps for years.

On the other hand, coming impotence often announces itself beforehand with certain well defined signals, such as diminishing vitality, decreasing frequency of desire, marked sexual apathy, lessening enjoyment.

Except for the impotency which arises out of serious chronic diseases or paralysis, the condition is one which in the vast majority of cases can be corrected. Impotency is not the natural lot of man- Nature never intended him to drag around a half-man, but intended that he should retain his all his life, be a full man, a strong man, a virile man, a potent man as long as life endured.

And there are countless instances of strong and vigorous old men of whom this condition is true; of men who have retained all the qualities of manhood to the end of long and useful careers, with mental factors in all vigor and alertness. Among the educated Hindus, as I have already said, this, indeed, is the common situation, impotency, so prevalent among us, the exception.

The regaining of lost manhood is an assured possibility, provided the right methods be followed. And right methods simmer down, really, to one right method, which is the method of the Hindus. There is no other plan or system or treatment which has ever shown that it can give better than temporary relief from the condition but the one which is practiced and advocated by the Hindus and which is being expounded by this course.

From time to time various methods are suggested, widely advertised and tried. Thirty years ago it was electricity. Electrical belts were sold by the millions. No good came of them. Then came pills and tablets, supposed in some mysterious way to stimulate the glands, give them a new surge of energy. All false. Right now expensive operations are widely touted as the cure for impotence and the restorer of vigor and virility. But even the most ardent advocates of operations admit that, in the majority of cases, the operations are doomed to failure at the start and that in the cases where they apparently succeed, their effect is temporary and must be renewed through successive operations in the future!

But while the rest of the world experimented and went up blind alleys in search of truth, the Hindu thinkers went blithely on their way, following age-old methods, and we have reached the point now where we can discover why these methods win while all others are so ineffective.

The secret is simple: the Hindu methods depend upon natural stimulation. All others depend upon unnatural stimulation. The 'Hindu methods depend upon continual stimulation; all others upon occasional stimulation. And there you have the difference in just a few words.

The Hindu belief, proved beyond doubt, is that when the body is reactivated, all the glands swing toward normal. When they get all the blood and natural stimulation they need, they perform their functions in a purely normal way. But unless conditions which reactivate the body are established, no lasting results can be hoped for from any artificial means.

The Hindu method of treating impotence and loss of virility is to show a man how to "operate" upon himself every day of his life, and thus rejuvenate and reactivate and stimulate those important glands and muscles and organs and procreative sources. '

Then he goes on year after year, his vital forces strong within him, young in body, young in mind, young in the vital forces which mean so much power and success in every field of human action.

Just exactly what these Hindu Secrets are you are now ready to learn, and in the next chapter they will be finally and fully revealed to you.

HINDU METHODS OF VIRILITY BUILDING

ALTHOUGH the basis of Hindu success in virility-building and rejuvenation is a regime of vital living, the cornerstone of the method is a series of simple body movements which are performed every day.

These movements are called *dands.*

They are the most amazing, most mysterious, most effective movements ever conceived for reactivating the entire body.

Please do not mistake them for physical culture or mere exercises, though they may resemble these. They are not exercises. They are scientific movements devised by skilled anatomists and are so far-reaching in their effects that they tend to recreate the person who uses them regularly.

And although they seem to be very simple, they are complex. No one mind could have conceived them, no one life could have perfected them. They are the result of the evolution of ages, and in their present form—just four simple movements—they will put into motion and gently stimulate and reactivate every muscle and organ and gland necessary in bringing about virility and rejuvenation.

The four movements must be done daily to have the desired effect. At first they must be done slowly and temperately, for they are vigorous in their influence and nothing is gained by strain. And the time required? At the outside five minutes a day.

isn't that a mighty cheap price to pay for so priceless a thing as virility?

Each of these movements serves a   purpose. The first, the Front Dand, stimulates the entire pelvic basin, the gonads, the thyroid, the thymus, the pituitary. The Reverse Dand stimulates all the procreative forces and reaches the lumbar region of the spine, while the third movement influences the hardening process of the abdominal walls, which, as you have learned, are so important in regaining and retaining virility. And the final movement is for the small of the back and all the procreative sources housed within the pelvic girdle.

These Hindu movements are not physical culture exercises and do not cause any strain. Anyone, regardless of age or condition, can use them, pro- vided he observes this warning: In the beginning, take it easy. Full directions for taking each movement, together with a progressive schedule, are given with the photographs of the movement. Follow this gentle plan in increasing the number of times you do   each Hindu movement, and there is going to be no ill effect.

If you want the best results you will go through the series in the morning, upon arising, and at night just before going to bed. It isn't necessary that you take the system twice a day, but it will bring about quicker results if you do. If you haven't time for the two a day schedule, go through the system either in the morning or at night.

Though the real Hindu secret consists of the use of these four Movements, the Hindus have discovered that other simple aids help in restoring virility.

Chief among these is cool water.

After going through the four Hindu Movements you should always take a Hindu natural bath. This is as simple to take as it is to describe:

Turn three to four inches of cool--not cold--water into the bathtub. It should be no cooler than 60° Fahrenheit. Sit in the tub, raise both knees and water over the abdomen, while you rub it vigorously with the hands and knead and pummel the entire abdominal region. Remain three minutes in the tub. No longer. Just before you get ready to step out, dip a sponge or towel in the water and the face, chest, spinal column and back of the neck.

Cool water produces a contraction of capillary blood vessels and more rapid circulation. It increases muscular tone, removes nervous irritability.

Warning: If you do not feel a warm glow of reaction after drying the body but instead feel it is a sign the water you are in the bath is too cold. Don't ever bathe in water too cold for comfort and swift reaction. Use warmer water. Water of 65°, 70°, even of 75° is Still cool enough have the intended effect, but it is better to keep it at 60° if you can.

The matter of diet is one which we can dispose of quickly. Diet in rebuilding or retaining virility is indeed important. But the diet which is required is, with certain minor alterations, so nearly like the normal diet everyone should eat that it can be easily described.

In the first place, one of the chief causes of lack of virility and impotency is chronic constipation.

Indeed, authorities say that they never saw a case 2 of impotency where constipation was not present. Therefore, one of the first things diet should do is to correct a condition of constipation.'

This is simpler than most persons realize. A normal diet, with plenty of bulky foods, with plenty of fruits, with a minimum of starchy concentrated foods, is the best cure, and a perfect preventive, of constipation.

If you suffer now from constipation, overhaul your diet so that you include more foods that give bulk and roughage—leafy vegetables (lettuce, spinach, cabbage and turnip greens, chard, broccoli, etc.), certain root vegetables eaten raw (carrots, turnips, etc.), fresh fruit and plenty of water—taken warm or cool, never iced.

This is the first step. The second is to drink each morning the juice of one lemon in a tumblerful of water and before each meal to take a tablespoonful of olive oil. At night eat an apple, and drink a glass of warm water just before going to bed.

Avoid cathartics, mineral oil, bran and all other medicines which are supposed to relieve constipation. Rely upon these simple natural methods. They never fail.

Eat fewer concentrated starchy foods, like white bread, pastry, cake. Keep sugar at a minimum.

Now for the virility—building diet.

Sexual apathy and impotence can almost always, as I have already indicated, be traced to depraved nutrition— which means some deficiency in diet. A diet deficient in iron, phosphorus, vitamins inhibits the normal secreting powers of the procreative sources. And how can you expect a finished product to be right if the raw materials of right quality and amount are not introduced into the factory?

The correction of depraved eating habits lies in eating food rich in the elements that go to build virility.

First of all this means that the diet should be rich in protein foods—lean meats, Fish, eggs, milk, butter. These invariably have an action upon the amative functions. The heads of spermatozoa, like the cell nuclei, consist of nucleo-proteins. When a considerable amount of food rich in nuclein is absorbed in the diet, the spermatozoa become more numerous and are apt to exert a normal exciting effect.

So in your diet make sure that you include a plentiful supply of eggs, meat, fish, milk, whole wheat bread and vegetables rich in iron and phosphorus, such as string beans, peas, lettuce, spinach, asparagus, cauliflower, celery.

Otherwise you may eat as you have been eating, for there is no good served in becoming a victim of some dietetic fad or in making a diet a fetish till you are afraid to eat this or that.

There are a few things which are harmful and which had better be minimized if not omitted. They are harmful when taken in excess; in normal quantities they probably do no harm. They are coffee, tea, alcoholic beverages and tobacco. It has been proved that if any of these is used in excess, it has the effect of diminishing vital power, rather than of increasing it. If you are using two cups of coffee a day, cut down to one; cut down on the others if you do not feel you want to cut them out entirely, which isn't at all necessary.

Chiefly you will get the benefit from these four marvelous Hindu Movements, and the next few pages describe these fully and show in picture exactly how each should be performed.

THE FIRST HINDU MOVEMENT

Rest the body on the hands and feet, hands about twenty-four inches apart, feet the same. Now arch the body so that the buttocks are as high in the air as you can get them.

Stretch, stretch and force and strain to reach higher with the buttocks. Make sure that the head is down and the chin is forced into the chest as shown by the illustration.

This is important, because of the effect it has on the important glands in the front of the neck.

Tense every muscle and hold for a second.

Now relax and permit the middle of the body to fall toward the floor but catch it, of course, before it actually strikes.

Now let the body come as close to the floor as it will without touching, and snap the head backward as far as it will go—a movement which influences the pituitary gland.

Stretch as far as you can and imagine you are lengthening the spine.

Tense the muscles.

Hold the position for a second and then raise the center of the body, lower the head and assume the top position of the movement.

This Front Dand was a very simple, very easy movement. But it has exerted a stimulating effect on the muscles surrounding the small of the back; it has stimulated the great 5 nerve centers, and it has caused a gentle stimulation to pass through all the procreative sources.

In the beginning do only two complete movements. Then adopt this scale of progression: The first week, 2 movements; the second week, 4; the third week, 8; the fourth week, 12; the fifth week, 16; the sixth week, 20. Hold at 20. That's enough to keep those muscles and glands stimulated and to reactivate them. Stand up for a rest between movements, put the hands on the hips and take two or three deep breaths. Then on to number two.

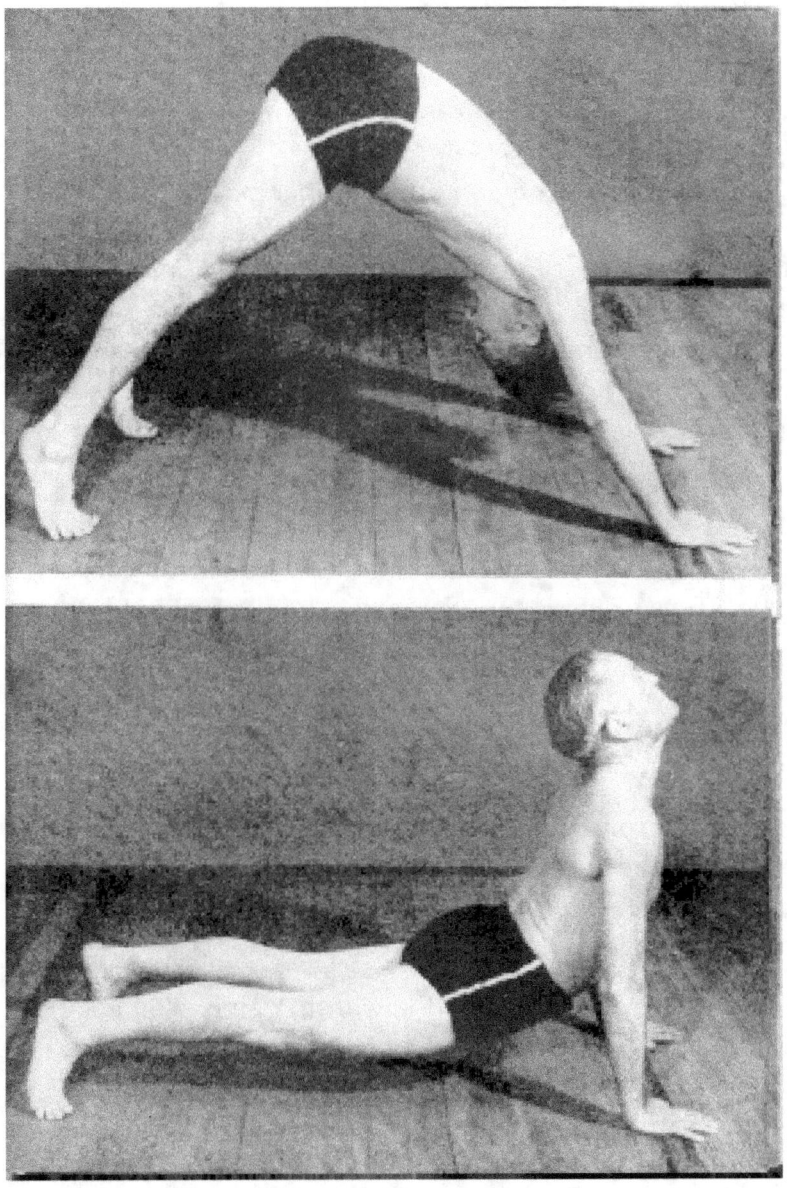

First Dand

THE SECOND HINDU MOVEMENT

The easiest way to assume the proper position for the Second Hindu Movement is to sit on the floor, then put the hands behind you, fingers facing away from the body, heels resting naturally on the floor. Now raise the buttocks off the Hoor slightly and force the chin hard against the chest.

This is the starting-point. Tense the muscles along the front the body and raise the abdomen as far as you can, as in the lower figure. As you come to the high point, relax the neck and force the head as far backward as you can, as shown. Tense every ·muscle in the body and hold the position for one second. Relax and come to the starting position. Hold there for a second. Raise again. This is a movement remarkable in its effect on the procreative sources.

Like the Front Dand it stimulates all the vital sources, reactivates the glands, tones up the muscles which surround the pelvic girdle and helps put you in good condition all over.

In the beginning abide by the warning given you about the First Hindu Movement: slow and easy. Start with two full counts. Then follow the regular progression table: 2 during the first week, 4 during the second, 8 during the third, 12 during the fourth, 16 during the fifth, 20 during the sixth.

And hold it there. Stand up for a moment of rest now, taking two or three deep breaths in front of the window. If, in the beginning, you have any sensation of breathlessness, stand still and breathe deeply until heart and lungs are functioning properly and normally before going to the Third Hindu Movement, which you will find described on the next page after the pictures of this Reverse Dand.

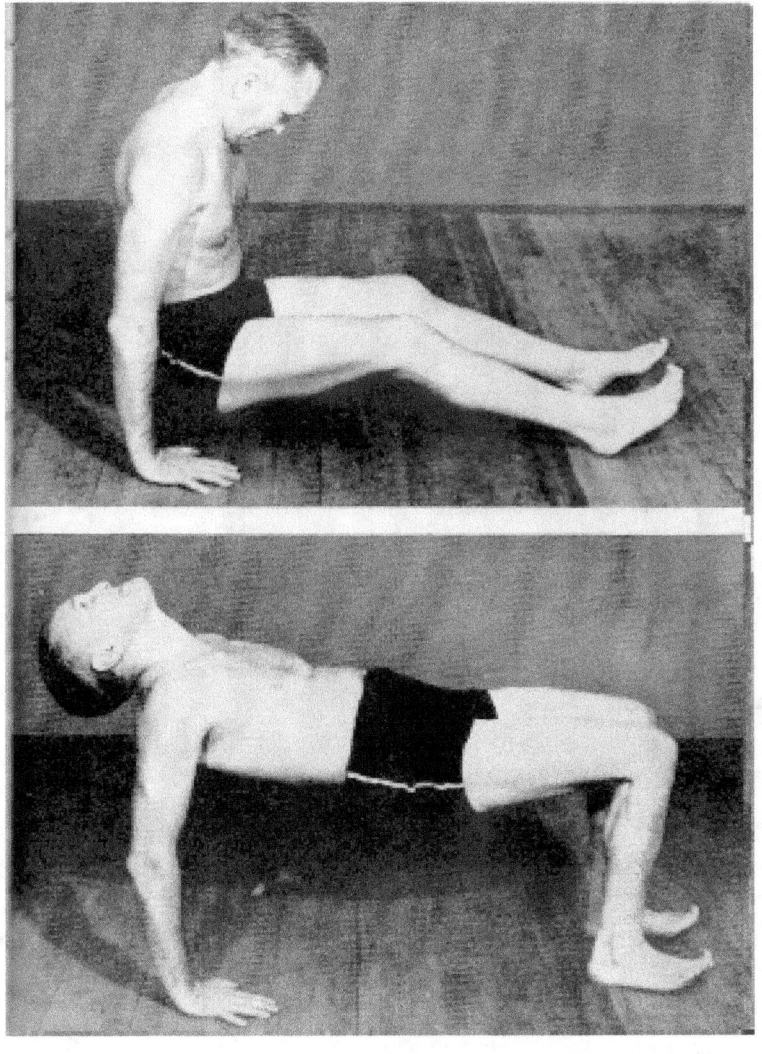

Second Dand

THE THIRD HINDU MOVEMENT

Primarily this simple movement cares for that distended abdomen from which so many men suffer and which is the cause of so much loss of vitality and virility. It is easy to perform, easier than the first two.

Lie on your back on the floor and put the hands, palms down, under the buttocks.

Now slowly raise the legs until they are perfectly vertical.

Hold them there for about a second and slowly let them to the floor. Don't relax and let them drop; keep control of them all the time. The region most affected by this Movement is the muscle sheath covering the lower abdomen. Perhaps in the beginning it will be too much for your softened muscles. Don't force them. If you find you haven't the strength to perform the movement, content yourself during the first two or three weeks with merely the legs at the knees and raising the knees toward the abdomen. If you suffer from hernia, better not try this at all in the more severe form, but rest content with the knee-raising version. And take it easy always, as you have advised. Raise the legs twice the first week; four times the second; then follow the regular progression: 8 movements in the third week; 12 in the fourth; 16, the fifth; 20, the sixth. Now get to your feet, and enjoy the sensation of two or three deep breaths before the open window. And on to Number Four.

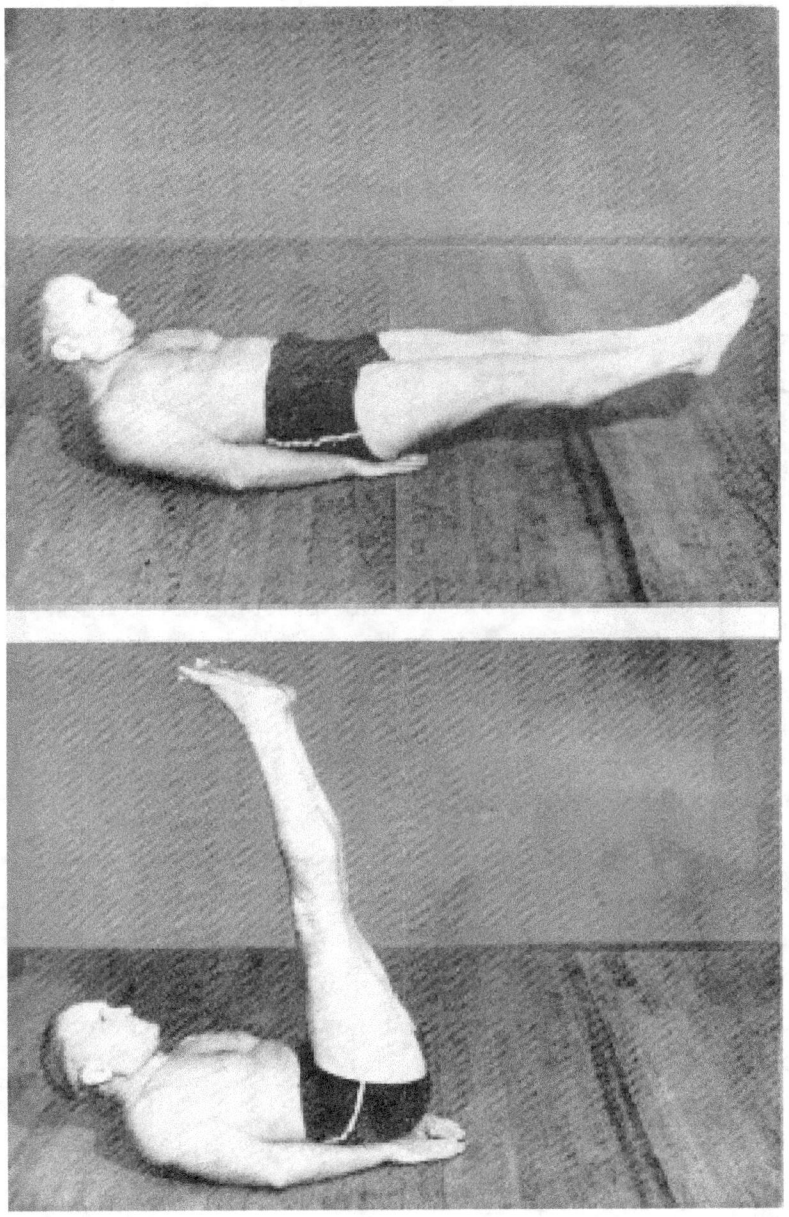

Third Dand

THE FOURTH HINDU MOVEMENT

There is not much action to this Hindu Movement, but it exerts a tremendously important effect nevertheless. Come to a kneeling position as shown. Place your hands, one on the back of each thigh. Hold the chest up, the body erect. This is the position at the start. The movement is very much restricted. Still holding the backs of the thighs, bend the body as far backward as you can. Come to the erect position. Bend back again. Now to the starting-position.

That is all there is to it, but it strengthens those spinal erector muscles that have so important a function in guarding vital nerve centers and procreative sources. Again you are warned: Take it easy. Two movements are enough the first week; 4 the second; 8 the third; 12 the fourth; 16 the fifth; 20 the sixth. It takes two minutes at the beginning, five minutes when you are doing more counts. And yet what a vast reward!

After you finish the Movements take the Hindu natural bath, dry yourself vigorously with a rough towel, and go about your business. Think nothing more of virility, rejuvenation. Lead a normal life. Enjoy whatever pleasures you like. Attend to your business. These simple Movements, plus directions for improving general physical condition, will begin building something fine, something very precious, something very wonderful into your system—the virility without which you are not a man!

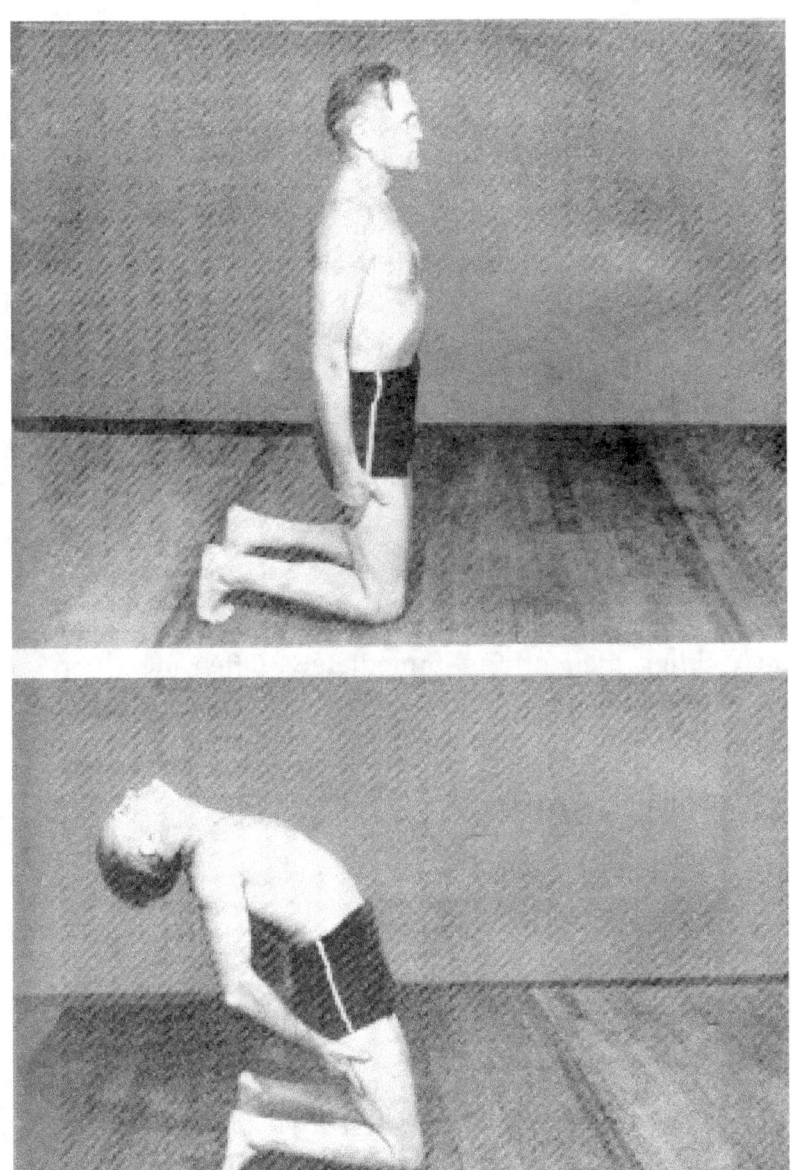

Fourth Dand

EPILOGUE. . .

AT THE BEGINNING of this course, I promised you that there would be nothing difficult, nothing complicated in these simple, but mysterious, Hindu Secrets of virility and rejuvenation.

Actually what is here only seems simple. In reality these Hindu Movements are almost as intricate and as complicated in their effect as the procreative forces themselves. They are put into simple form, but their influence reaches every organ, every gland, every muscle, every nerve which in any way influences the priceless heritage of virility.

And the most fascinating thing about them is that they begin yielding their profits immediately. Often men who begin these Movements tell me that they notice results at once, the very next day.

What will be the results?

The first one which you will notice will be an improvement in the way you feel. You will feel better all over, younger, more resilient physically and mentally. Your weariness will disappear. You will work longer. You will be less fatigued.

Intestinal disturbances, so common with men of thirty-Eve or over, will disappear. You will sleep better. Your meals will taste better. In short, you'll be a different man. And gradually you will notice an improvement in those procreative sources which are so important to your well-being. Youthful enthusiasm will be restored. The powers which have been waning in your life for months, perhaps for years, will return to you, and then will come the satisfaction of life which only men who are whole men can feel.

Behind these practices, as you have learned, lie 2,000 years of philosophy and scholarly research and Hindu culture; behind you as you practice them are also the lives of millions of men who, by following the road upon which you have set out, have lived full and complete and happy lives of strength and satisfaction and abiding health.

Your feet are on the road now to some of the finest favors which life can grant.

Good luck attend you at every step!

(This concludes the original Emil Raux text.)

VI

SEMINAL NUTRITION

While *The Hindu Secrets of Virility & Rejuvenation* provides a general overview of preferred dietary practices, the ensuing 75 years has yielded a great deal further wisdom on how best to nourish the body for fertility. And while not meant to be comprehensive treatise on nutrition, the powerful botanicals and superfoods shared in this section will have the effect of greatly enhancing one's virility.

FLOWER POWER—FERTILITY FUEL FROM THE BEEHIVE

By far and away the best single supplement known for the restoration of male seminal power is bee pollen, a soft granulated powder with a mildly sweet flavor. On a broader systemic level, it has been demonstrated to routinely improve the performance of even peak-condition Olympic athletes by an average of 15%.

"A DUD AT 70—A STUD AT 80"—THE RESURRECTION OF NOEL JOHNSON

The power of bee pollen is borne out in the life of Noel Johnson—who, at the age of 65, was a smoker, overweight, with a heart on the brink of failing.

He also found himself impotent—lacking libido and incapable of erection.

Due to these infirmities, he was turned down for life insurance and given six months to live, and advised by his physicians to refrain even from mowing his lawn.

But Johnson refused to accept this prognosis and opted to radically change his lifestyle. He began walking and cultivating a more healthful diet. Bee pollen featured prominently in his supplementation program, and, within a relatively short period, he was running regularly. He became fit and healthy again.

From this time on, he became a zealous athletic competitor, running 21 marathons, setting world records for seniors in the New York marathon, and also holding a boxing record as the World's Greatest Senior Boxer.

Equally gratifying was that he also recovered his virility, and went on to enjoy several late life romances, which he directly attributes to the strange golden granules.

While enthusiastic about many health supplements, Johnson attributes his success overwhelmingly to his use of bee pollen, confirming, "I made the use of bee pollen the essential facet of my nutrition program ..."

He discovered bee pollen to be a concentrated source of minerals, vitamins, proteins, amino acids and enzymes – a powerhouse of critical nutrients. It is, in fact, the only substance which is known to contain almost every known nutrient.

Noel Johnson went on to write two books on the story of his comeback, *Living Proof: I Have Found the Fountain of Youth* and *A Dud at 70, A Stud at 80: How To Do It.*

He passed at the ripe old age of 96, having lived a full and passionate life.

Pollen is the male seed of flowers, required for the fertilization of the plant. The tiny particles consist of 50/1,000-millimeter corpuscles, formed at the free end of the stamen in the heart of the blossom. Every variety of flower puts forth a dusting of pollen, as do many orchard fruits and agricultural food crops.

Bee pollen is the food of the young bee and it is approximately 40% protein. Considered one of nature's most completely nourishing foods, it contains nearly all nutrients required by humans. About half of its protein is in the form of free amino acids that are ready to be used directly by the body. Such highly assimilable protein can contribute significantly to one's protein needs.

One of the most intriguing facts about bee pollen is that it cannot be synthesized in a laboratory. When researchers remove a bee's natural comb-pollen and feed her manmade pollen, the bee dies even though all the known nutrients are present in the lab-synthesized product. While many thousands of chemical analyses of bee pollen have been done, there still remain some elements present that science cannot identify. The bees add some mysterious alchemy of their own, unidentifiable elements may contain the clue as to why bee pollen works so spectacularly against so many diverse conditions of ill health.

A one teaspoon dose of pollen takes one bee working eight hours a day for one month to gather! Each bee pollen pellet contains over two million flower pollen grains and one teaspoonful contains over 2.5 billion grains of flower pollen.

Complete Nutrition

Bee pollen contains all the essential components of life. The percentage of rejuvenating elements in bee pollen, remarkably, exceeds even those present in brewer's yeast and wheat germ. By covering such a complete spectrum of nutrients, bee pollen corrects nutritional deficiencies created by the unbalanced nutrition so rampant in the present world, relying as it does upon industrialized, processed and fragmented foods, often laden with thousands of chemicals.

Pollen is considered an energy and nutritive tonic in Chinese medicine. Cultures throughout the world use it in a surprising number of applications, among them:

Improving endurance and vitality

Extending longevity

Aiding recovery from chronic illness

Adding weight during convalescence

Reducing cravings and addictions

Building new blood

Helping overcome retardation and other developmental problems in children

Preventing infectious diseases such as the cold and flu (it has antibiotic type properties)

Pollen is also thought to protect against radiation and to have anti-cancer qualities.

Because bee pollen contains all the nutrients needed to sustain life, it is being used on an ever-larger scale for human nourishment and health. There are numerous reports from medical experience that conclusively show the benefits of bee pollen exceed that of a simple food item. And the bees do most of the work.

Bee-gathered pollens are rich in proteins, free amino acids, and vitamins, including B-complex and folic acid.

According to researchers at the Institute of Apiculture, Taranov, Russia:

"Honeybee pollen is the richest source of vitamins found in nature in a single food. Even if bee pollen had none of its other vital ingredients, its content of rutin alone would justify taking at least a teaspoon daily, if for no other reason than strengthening the capillaries. Pollen is extremely rich in rutin and may have the highest content of any source, plus it provides a high content of the nucleics RNA [ribonucleic acid] and DNA [deoxyribonucleic acid]."

Bee pollen is a complete food and contains many elements that products of animal origin do not possess. It is richer in proteins than any animal source, and contains more amino acids than beef, eggs, or cheese of equal weight. Bee pollen is particularly concentrated in all elements necessary for life.

Medical Miracles

Researchers have demonstrated that there is a substance in bee pollen that inhibits the development of numerous harmful bacteria. Experiments have shown bee pollen contains an antibiotic factor effective against salmonella and some strains of bacteria. Clinical studies have shown that it exerts a regulatory effect on intestinal function. The presence of a high proportion of cellulose and fiber in pollen, as well as the existence of antibiotic factors, all contribute to an explanation for this effectiveness.

Tests upon lab animals has demonstrated that the ingestion of bee pollen has a good effect on the composition of blood. A considerable and simultaneous increase of both white and red blood cells is observed. When bee pollen is given to anemic patients, their levels of hemoglobin (oxygen-carrying red blood cells) increase considerably.

It is reported that bee pollen in the diet acts to normalize cholesterol and triglyceride levels in the blood: upon the regular ingestion of bee pollen, a reduction of cholesterol and triglycerides was observed. High-density lipoproteins (HDL) increased, while low-density lipoproteins (LDL) decreased. A normalization of blood serum cholesterol levels is also seen.

One of the most important articles ever published on bee pollen comes from the United States Department of Agriculture (USDA). This article, titled "Delay in the Appearance of Palpable Mammary Tumors in C3H Mice Following the Ingestion of Pollenized Food," is the work of William Robinson of the Bureau of Entomology, Agriculture Research Administration. It was published in the *Journal of the National Cancer Institute* way back in October 1948, five decades ago. According to the article, Dr. Robinson started with mice that had been specially bred to develop and subsequently die from tumors. He explains, "The age at which mice of this strain developed tumors ranged from 18 to 57 weeks, with an average appearance at 33 weeks. Tumor incidence was 100 percent."

The pollen used in this study was supplied by the Division of Bee Culture and, according to the report, "was the bee-gathered type." One group of mice was fed mice chow only; another group was fed mice chow with the addition of bee pollen at a ratio of 1 part bee pollen to 10,000 parts food. Dr. Robinson's article states:

"Particular attention was given to the weight of the treated animals, since underweight can in itself bring about a delay in tumor development. No decrease in weight occurred in the animals receiving the pollenized food. Instead, a slight but fairly uniform increase was noted, possibly due to a nutritional factor in pollen."

In his summary, Dr. Robinson reveals the dramatic results:

"In the untreated mice [the mice not given bee pollen], mammary tumors appeared as expected at an average of 31.3 weeks. Tumor incidence was 100 percent. In the postponement series, [the mice given bee pollen], the average [onset of tumors] was 41.1 weeks, a delay of 9.8 weeks being obtained. Seven mice in this series were still tumor-free at 56 to 62 weeks of age, when the tests were terminated. I would like to emphasize that these mice were especially bred to die from cancerous tumors. Without the protection of bee pollen in their food, the mice developed tumors and died right on schedule."

Given the fact that cancer is the number-two killer in the United States (heart disease is number one), we can all certainly agree that this is an electrifying article. What happened from it? Nothing. Even the National Cancer Institute, which published it, failed to follow up on this very promising line of research. It was dropped with no explanation.

More good news comes from the University of Vienna, where Dr. Peter Hernuss and colleagues conducted a study of 25 women suffering from inoperable uterine cancer. Because surgery was impossible, the women were treated with chemotherapy. The lucky women given bee pollen with their food quickly exhibited a higher concentration of cancer-fighting immune-system cells, increased antibody production, and a markedly improved level of infection-fighting and oxygen carrying red blood cells (hemoglobin). These women suffered less from the awful side effects of chemotherapy as well. Bee pollen lessened the terrible nausea that commonly accompanies the treatment and helped keep hair loss to a minimum. The women also slept better at night. The control group receiving a placebo did not experience comparable relief.

A report from the Agronomic Institute, Faculty of Zootechnics, Romania, showed the immune-strengthening effects of bee pollen. According to the report "Comparative Studies Concerning Biochemical Characteristics of Beebread as Related to the Pollen Preserved in Honey" by Drs. E. Palos, Z. Voiculescu, and C. Andrei:

"An increase has been recorded in the level of blood lymphocytes, gamma globulins, and proteins in those subjects given pollen in comparison with control groups. The most significant difference occurred in lymphocytes. These results thus signify a strengthening in the resistance of the organic system."

Lymphocytes are the white blood cells that are the "soldiers" of the immune system. They are responsible for ridding the body of injurious and harmful substances, including infected or diseased cells, mutant and cancerous cells, viruses, metabolic trash, and so on. Gamma globulin is a protein formed in the blood, and our ability to resist infection is closely related to this protein's activity.

Infertility Problems

Pollen stimulates ovarian function. The best results were obtained with a pollen supplementation of 2 parts per 100 in the ration, and with the substitution of animal proteins with pollen in a proportion of 5 parts per 100. The intensity of ovulation increased. Parallel to this increase in ovulation, pollen also improves the ability of eggs to withstand the incubation period. The best results were obtained with a quantity of 4 parts per 100 of pollen added to the ration, resulting in an increase in the percentage of eggs in respect to the control group. The application of pollen is recommended whenever the end result is obtaining eggs for reproduction.

Bee Products Also Treats Allergies!

Pollen is also a remedy for hay fever and allergies. However, it must be taken at least six weeks before the season begins and then continued throughout the season if it going to work.

Bee pollen has been effectively used down through the ages to rid allergy sufferers of their afflictions. This technique, called desensitization, was developed at St. Mary's Hospital Medical School in London soon after the turn of the century. The treatment consists of administering small amounts of the allergen to stimulate the patient's own immune system to produce antibodies that will eliminate the allergic reaction. It works rather like a vaccination does against childhood diseases.

Desensitization is based on the premise that the administration of the allergen will cause the body to produce antibodies that will cancel out the effects of the offending substance when the patient is again exposed to it.

Leo Conway, M.D., of Denver Colorado, treated his patients with pollen. Dr. Conway reported: "All patients who had taken the antigen [pollen] for three years remained free from all allergy symptoms, no matter where they lived and regardless of diet. Control has been achieved in 100 percent of my earlier cases and the field is ever-expanding." Since oral feeding of pollen for this use was first perfected in his laboratory, astounding results were obtained. No ill consequences have resulted. Ninety-four percent of all his patients were completely free from allergy symptoms. Of the other six percent, not one followed directions, but even this small percentage were nonetheless partially relieved.

Relief of hay fever, pollen-induced asthma, with ever increasing control of bronchitis, ulcers of the digestive tract, colitis, migraine headaches, and urinary disorders were all totally successful. Unfortunately, Dr. Conway, an early pioneer in the field of allergies, is now deceased. What we did not know was just how lightning-fast it could bring relief. It actually eliminated longstanding symptoms in minutes. Everything from asthma to allergies to sinus problems cleared. These trials confirmed that bee pollen is wonderfully effective against a very wide range of respiratory distress.

Bee Products and Physical Activity

The British Sports Council recorded increases in strength of as high as 40 to 50 percent in those taking bee pollen regularly. Even more astounding, the British Royal Society has reported height increases in adults who take pollen.

Antii Lananaki, coach of the Finnish track team that swept the Olympics in 1972, revealed, "Most of our athletes take pollen food supplements. Our studies show it significantly improves their performance. There have been no negative results since we have been supplying pollen to our athletes."

Alex Woodly, then executive director of the prestigious Education Athletic Club in Philadelphia, said:

"Bee pollen works, and it works perfectly. Pollen allows super-stars to increase their strength and stamina up to 25 percent. This increase in strength and endurance may be the key to the secret regenerative power of bee pollen. Bee pollen causes a definite decrease in pulse rate. The whole beauty of bee pollen is that it's as natural as you can get. No chemicals. No steroids."

Renowned German naturalist Francis Huber was a great proponent of this miraculous food from the hive. Huber called bee pollen "the greatest body builder on Earth."

Bee Pollen and Weight Control

Bee pollen works wonders in a weight-control or weight-stabilization regimen by correcting a possible chemical imbalance in body metabolism that may be involved in either abnormal weight gain or loss. The normalizing and stabilizing effects of this perfect food from the bees are phenomenal.

In weight-loss programs, bee pollen stimulates the metabolic processes. It speeds caloric burn by lighting and stoking the metabolic fires. Honeybee pollen is coming to be recognized as Nature's true weight-loss food. Bee pollen is a low-calorie food. It contains only ninety calories per ounce. (An ounce is about two heaping tablespoons.) It offers 15 percent lecithin by volume.

Lecithin is a substance that helps dissolve and flush fat from the body. This is one reason why bee pollen lowers low-density lipoproteins (LDL) surer and faster than any other food while helping increase the helpful high-density lipoproteins (HDL), which science says protect against cholesterol and heart disease.

Chemistry notes that honeybee pollen contains potent antibiotics that can act to reverse the effects normal aging exerts on skin, correcting darkening, wrinkles, and blemishes.

Some further insights on bee pollen, extrapolated from an article by Govan Kilgour, follow:

Bee pollen is an alkaline food that balances the overall pH of your body. Most researchers agree that its nutritional profile is one of the most complete in the world. It can be used as an alternative to a multivitamin.

Contents in Bee Pollen:

25% to 40% vegetarian complete protein (in pre-digested, free amino acid form)

A variety of fatty acids (70% is the omega 3 *ALA*, 3-4% is the Omega 6 *LA* and 16-17% is monounsaturated and saturated fat)

Simple carbohydrates (many of the same sugars that are found in honey.)

All the B vitamins (including biotin, folic acid, choline and inositol but not a usable form of B12)

Vitamin C

Vitamin D (which is rare for plant foods to contain)

Vitamin E

Vitamin K

Up to 60 major and minor minerals (including some rare elements like gold in amounts as high as 0.9 parts per million depending on the type of flower pollen used).

Nucleic acids such as RNA and DNA (a component found in the diets of many centenarians).

Steroidal and hormonal substances (natural plant sources of these are safe and beneficial).

15% lecithin (dissolves cholesterol plaque and a potent food for the brain).

High on the ORAC (Oxygen Radical Absorption Capacity) scale due to a wide array of antioxidants (it is scored at 164, while blueberries are a 61).

Rutin (a key antioxidant for strengthening the walls of the vascular system, also helps stabilize vitamin C)

Carotenoids such as xanthophyll and alpha/beta carotenes (the more antioxidant carotenoids a mammal gets, the longer it can live).

At least 11 major enzymes (which are necessary for digestion. Bee pollen benefits and complements a live food diet since the extra enzymes have an anti-aging effect on the cells of the body).

Over 5000 minor enzymes and coenzymes (arguably the most enzyme rich substance in existence).

1-3% of pollen is made up of unidentified "mysterious" compounds, very possibly highly valuable Ormus minerals.

It takes one bee working eight hours a day, one month to gather a single teaspoon of bee pollen granules. But that teaspoon of bee pollen granules contains 2.5 billion grains of flower pollen.

The performance of even world-class Olympic athletes routinely improves as much as 15% when bee pollen is added to their daily regimen. Antti Lananaki who was the coach of the Finish track team that swept the Olympics in 1972, revealed, "most of our athletes take pollen food supplements. Our studies show it significantly improves their performance. There have been no negative results since we have been supplying pollen to our athletes." Some bee pollen studies done in Britain by the British Sports Council recorded increases in strength as much as 40% to 50% in those getting the benefits of taking bee pollen. The British Royal Society has even reported height increases in *adults* who regularly take bee pollen granules!

Over 40 bee pollen studies have confirmed bee pollen to be safe to consume and that it even has therapeutic effects. Bee pollen benefits the body virtually instantly; the granules pass through the lining of the stomach into the bloodstream, and within 2 hours it can even be found in the cerebrospinal fluid!

For centuries, it has been a dietary staple for longevity.

Apart from its benefits to athletes, pollen offers documented help in reversing the following conditions:

Acne
Allergies
Anemia
Asthma
Bronchitis
Constipation
Colitis
Obesity
Relief of symptoms of type 2 diabetes
Sinusitis
Wrinkles

It was found that the high numbers of super-centenarians in "The Garden of Eden in Caucasus" (mountains of Abkhazia) seemed to have an affinity for consuming bee pollen, royal jelly and raw honey products on a daily basis.

Nicholai Tsitsin, a Russian biologist, published a report in 1945 on 150 Russian centenarians who returned questionnaires about their diet, age and occupation and he found that *all* of them consumed hive products. It was specifically the "left over" raw honey scrapings from the bottom of the hive where the bee pollen granules fell to the bottom and got mixed in that they consumed.

After physical examinations, Dr. Tsitin discovered that bee pollen benefits the centenarians through heart attack protection. Many of them had signs and scars of "silent heart attacks", which he determined would have killed anyone at an earlier age who didn't have the protective benefits of taking bee pollen.

It is interesting to note that the natives of the Caucasus region of Russia were known to eat a predominantly plant based diet that also contained a significant amount of raw living foods such as fruits, vegetables, nuts and seeds. When this is combined with the consumption of bee pollen, the body is provided with an abundance of all the necessary enzymes needed to digest food, while avoiding tapping into the body's natural store of metabolic enzymes.

A reasonable starting dose would be from ½ to 1 teaspoon twice a day, straight or blended into drinks, moving up to a teaspoon 2 or even 3 times per day. For extreme physical—or, as it may happen, sexual—activity these doses may be doubled and even tripled.

MACA MAGIC

Maca is both an herb and a food of Peruvian origin, long revered for its ability to restore sexual vitality.

Psychiatrist and functional medicine physician Hyla Cass, MD, says maca works. "In my practice, I have seen maca restore hormonal imbalance and related sexual desire and fertility in both men and women."

Christopher Kilham, author of *Hot Plants*, says, "Maca enjoys a very long history of successful medicinal use for menopausal discomfort, infertility, and sexual healing. The question is not whether it works—because we know it works with certainty—but *how* it works."

The remainder of this chapter, further revealing the powers of maca, is excerpted from *Maca Restores Sexual Health without Raising Hormone Levels*, by Barbara L. Minton, published on the *Natural News* website.

Inca warriors knew maca could increase their stamina, and they ate the root before going into battle. Maca also increased their sexual health and virility. Legend has it that maca was kept from the warriors when they returned from battle to protect the women.

Today, scientists in Italy have documented the ability of maca to increase general and sexual well-being in patients with mild erectile dysfunction (ED). In a double-blind clinical trial using 50 men affected by mild ED, half received maca dry extract at 2,400 mg, and the other half received a placebo. Treatment effect and subjective well-being were measured before and after 12 weeks. Both the maca treated men and those receiving the placebo experienced a significant increase in their erectile function scores and on scores revealing improvement in psychological performance. However, the scores of the maca treated group were significantly higher than the placebo group. Only the maca treated patients experienced a significant improvement in physical and social performance compared with their baseline scores. (*Andrologia*, April)

Researchers at Massachusetts General Hospital studied maca for its effect on selective serotonin reuptake inhibitor (SSRI) induced sexual dysfunction. They conducted a double-blind study comparing a low dose (1.5 g/day) to a high-dose (3.0 g/day) maca regimen in 20 depressed outpatients with SSRI induced sexual dysfunction. Patients receiving the higher dose showed a significant improvement on a sexual experience scale and sexual function questionnaire, while subjects on the lower dose did not. Libido improved significantly and was not differentiated by dose amount. Maca was well tolerated by both groups. (*CNS Neuroscience*, Fall, 2008).

These studies followed groundbreaking research done by scientists in Peru who in 2002 treated 56 healthy male subjects ages 21 to 56 years with maca. They sought to determine whether the effect of maca was the result of change in mood or in serum testosterone levels. The men received 1,500 mg or 3,000 mg of maca, or a placebo. An improvement in sexual desire was observed by week 8 of treatment. Serum testosterone and estradiol levels were no different in men treated with maca than in those treated with placebo. However, measures of sexual desire increased by 42.2% in the group taking the higher dose. Analysis revealed that maca has an independent effect on sexual desire that is not the result of changes in mood or hormone levels. (*Andrologia*, December, 2002).

Maybe the best thing about maca is that it does not work like synthetic ED drugs that produce hormonal changes that may lead to unwanted side effects. Maca has been shown not to change testosterone levels. (*Phytomedicine*, August, 2007).

Among doctors using maca in their practice to treat the symptoms of ED, male impotence and menopause are Doctor Aquila Calderon, past dean of the National University of Federico Villareal Faculty of Human Medicine, and Dr. Gary Gordon, past president of the American College for Advancement in Medicine in Arizona.

Maca reduces psychological symptoms in women without raising hormone levels.

Maca is also good for what ails women, but does not alter their hormone status. Researchers in Australia examined the estrogenic and androgenic activity of maca and its effect on the hormonal profiles and symptoms of postmenopausal women. Fourteen women were given 3.5 g/day of powered maca or a matching placebo for 6 weeks. Blood samples were assessed to determine steroid hormone levels. No differences were seen between baseline, maca treatment, and placebo treatment in serum concentrations of estradiol, follicle-stimulating hormone, luteinizing hormone, or sex hormone-binding globulin. However, findings showed that maca significantly reduced psychological symptoms, including anxiety and depression, and lowered measures of sexual dysfunction. (*Menopause*, November-December, 2008).

Maca was shown effective at preventing hormone related bone loss. Scientist in China evaluated an extract of maca on induced postmenopausal osteoporosis in rats. Bone mineral density and histopathological parameters indicated maca was able to prevent bone loss resulting from estrogen deficiency. (*Journal of Ethnopharmacology*, April 21, 2006).

Maca is both a food and an herb

The most active part of maca is its starchy, tuberous root, which is referred to as an herb, but maca is actually a food from the cruciferous vegetable family. In looks it resembles the radish, but in taste it is more like the potato. Like wheat and rice, maca contains protein, fats, carbohydrates, and dietary fiber. It is rich in magnesium, selenium and calcium, and fatty acids.

Maca is grown at high elevation in the Andes, and the plant requires very cold climate and high altitudes to achieve maximum potency. Not all varieties of maca on the market have been grown under ideal conditions.

Maca is a classic adaptogen

Adaptogens are substances that raise the non-specific resistance in an organism. They enable it to adapt to external conditions and work with its own natural rhythms to help rebuild systems and restore homeostasis. The ancient Andes mountain dwellers knew about the adaptogenic properties of maca and its ability to keep the body on an even keel. Folk medicine tradition describes how maca helped highlanders thrive at altitudes of 14,000 to 18,000 feet above sea level where oxygen content in the blood is low.

Modern scientists and doctors have found maca to be one of the best natural ways to regulate and support the endocrine system. Through this action, energy levels, metabolism, growth, sexual development, and psychology are normalized.

In today's world, adaptogens such as maca take on a greater significance than in the past, because of constantly increasing levels of stress. Dr. Hans Seyle, Nobel Prize winning author of several works on adaptation, was the first to demonstrate the existence of biological stress. He described how the human body adapts to stress, and the stages it passes through when the stress goes unmitigated. He pointed out that positive or negative, stress is still stress and it differs from all other physical responses.

The system whereby the body copes with stress, the hypothalamic-pituitary axis (HPA axis) system, was first described by Selye. He pointed to an "alarm state", a "resistance state", and an "exhaustion state", largely referring to glandular states. Later he developed the idea of two "reservoirs" of stress resistance, or what he referred to as "alternative" stress energy.

Maca works to effectively help the body adapt to the high levels of stress involved in modern living. This adaptive mechanism involves normalization of both men's and women's hormonal imbalances. Instead of supplying plant hormones such as phytoestrogens, maca acts on the HPA pathway that is the precursor of male and female hormones. It also has an effect on the adrenal glands. Maca does not necessarily stimulate, but acts in a regulatory fashion balancing and returning homeostasis.

Maca helps normalize learning and memory too. Researchers from China studied the effect of black maca on learning and memory in hormonally deprived rats. They found that experimental memory impairments induced by hormonal deprivation were reduced in rats given black maca, due in part to its antioxidant activities. (*Evidenced Based Complementary Alternative Medicine*, October 9, 2000).

Maca shows remarkable ability to reduce prostate enlargement

Maca has demonstrated its ability to affect the size of the prostate according to seasoned researchers of maca in Lima, Peru. Their study was designed to determine the effect of red maca in prostate enlargement induced with a testosterone hormone drug in adult mice. Mice were examined at intervals during treatment. Testosterone and estradiol were assessed on the last day of treatment. The researchers found that red maca reduced prostate weight at 21 days of treatment. Weights of the seminal vesicle, testis and epididymis were not affected by the treatment. (*Andrologia*, June, 2008).

Maca shown to increase sperm count

Meanwhile, another research group in Lima evaluated the effect of different fractions of black maca on sperm creation. Maca was given along with one of several solvents. The greatest increase in sperm creation occurred in the group given the ethyl acetate fraction from the black maca extract, suggesting that the compounds related to the beneficial effect on sperm production of black maca are presented in this fraction. What can be fractioned out with a solvent is there in the maca totality, so males eating maca may expect some of this beneficial result. (*Fertility Sterility*, May, 2008).

Using maca

The maca vegetable appears in health food stores occasionally. It has a sweet taste and can be eaten in a number of ways including raw, dried, baked or boiled. In Peru cookies, tarts and even mixed drinks are made with maca. Most consumers in the U.S. will have access to maca only as a supplement in the form of an extract, whole root herb, or as gelatinized root.

As a general rule, the gelatinized form has the highest level of bioavailability. Gelatinization does not refer to the presence of gelatin or that it is enclosed in a gelatin capsule. It is actually a process that removes the starch from the maca root and breaks down the chemical bonds that connect the starch to the protein and other components. With maca that is ungelatinized, the body must do the processing in the digestive tract, as preferred by people who shun excessive processing. A source of gelatinized maca root is the National University of Agriculture at La Molina, Peru.

There is red, yellow and black maca. Each seems to have a unique component for addressing sexual health. Black maca has been shown to be the most beneficial variety for reducing ED, for increasing sperm count and sperm motility, and for restoring learning and memory. Red maca is the variety most associated with reducing prostate size.

THINK ZINC

The importance of zinc in prostate health cannot be overestimated, as evidenced by the following research conclusions (Life Extension Magazine, 2015):

Prostate cancer remains the second most common malignancy in men, after skin cancer, and the second leading cause of cancer death, after lung cancer.

The trace metal zinc plays a unique role in prostate health; the prostate gland accumulates zinc at 10 to 15 times higher concentration than other body tissues.

Zinc helps prostate cells resist malignant transformation by creating an intracellular environment toxic to cancerous cells; normal prostate cells have evolved powerful mechanisms to protect themselves against zinc toxicity.

Basic laboratory studies reveal potent effects of prostate cell zinc content on fundamental cancer-promoting properties of cells.

Men over 40 should consider zinc supplementation for a variety of reasons including maintaining healthy prostate tissue zinc levels.

The following foods are rich in zinc—so critical to prostate health, and have long been traditional staples in native diets for support of sexual function.

HIGH ZINC FOODS
  pumpkin seeds
  squash seeds
  sesame seeds
  egg yolks
  kidney beans
  lima beans
  chickpeas
  flax seeds
  garlic
  mushrooms
  shellfish (oysters, shrimp, clams, lobster,etc.)

VII

TAOIST REJUVENATION TECHNIQUE:
THE MALE DEER ENERGY EXERCISE

The following exercise is a time-honored—and, quite literally, hands-on—practice for re-energizing the sexual anatomy and constitutes a valuable adjunct for anyone wishing to maximize his vitality. (With thanks to, and as described by, Dr. Stephen Chang in *The Tao of Sexology*, Tao Publishing, 1986)

The Male Deer Exercise achieves four important objectives. First, it builds up the tissues of the sexual organs. Second, it draws energy up through six of the Seven Glands of the body into the pineal gland to elevate spirituality. (There is a hormone pathway that leads from the prostate, connects with the adrenal glands, and continues on to the other glands.) Concurrently, blood circulation in the abdominal area is increased. This rush of blood helps transport the nutrients and energy of the semen to the rest of the body.

When energy is brought up into the pineal gland, a chill or tingling sensation is felt to ascend through the spine to reach the head. It feels a little like an orgasm. If you feel a sensation in the area of the pineal gland, but do not feel the tingling sensation in the middle of the back, do not worry. Your sensitivity will increase with experience. If after some time you still cannot sense the progress of energy, certain problems must be taken care of first.

Self-determination is the third benefit derived from the Deer Exercise. If one gland in the Seven Gland system is functioning below par, the energy shooting up the spine will stop there. A weakness is indicated, and special attention should be given to that area. For example, if the thymus gland is functioning poorly, the energy will stop there. The energy will continue to stop there until the thymus gland is healed. When the thymus is again functioning normally, the energy will then move further up along the spine toward the pineal gland. If the energy moves all the way up to your head during the Deer Exercise, it indicates that all the Seven Glands are functioning well and that there is no energy blockage in the body,. If you do not feel anything during the Deer Exercise, a blockage is indicated. The movement of energy can be felt by everyone if no dysfunctions are encountered.

The fourth benefit of the Deer Exercise is that it builds up sexual ability and enables the man to prolong sexual intercourse. During "ordinary" intercourse the prostate swells with semen to maximum size before ejaculating. During ejaculation, the prostate shoots out its contents in a series of contractions. Then, sexual intercourse ends. With nothing left to ejaculate, induce contractions, or maintain an erection (energy is lost during ejaculation), the man cannot continue to make love. But, if he uses the Deer Exercise to pump semen out of the prostate in small doses, pumping it in the other direction into the other glands and blood vessels, he can prolong intercourse.

Under ordinary circumstances, when the Deer Exercise is not used during intercourse, it will be harmful to interrupt orgasm or prolong intercourse by ordinary means. Under ordinary means, the prostate remains expanded for a long time, unrelieved by the pumping action of the ejaculation, until the semen is carried away by the blood stream. But the prostate is somewhat like a rubber band: it must be allowed to snap back to its original form, otherwise continuous extension will bring about a loss of elasticity. When the prostate loses its elasticity, its function is impaired and it is damaged. The Deer Exercise prolongs orgasm and intercourse, but it protects the prostate by relieving it.

The Deer Exercise is a physical exercise as well as a mental and spiritual exercise. It improves one's sexual abilities as it builds up the energy reserves within the body. Over time, the mental processes are heightened as well, and the outcome is often a glowing feeling of inner tranquility, which is a necessary prerequisite for the unfolding of the golden flower.

This exercise may be done standing, sitting, or lying down.

First Stage —

The purpose of the first stage is to encourage semen production.

Rub the palms of your hands together vigorously. This creates heat in your hands by bringing the energy of your body into your hands and palms.

With your right hand, cup your testicles so that the palm of your hand completely covers them. (The exercise is best done without clothing.) Do not squeeze, but apply a slight pressure, and be aware of the heat from your hand.

Place the palm of your left hand on the area of the pubis, one inch below the navel.

With a slight pressure so that a gentle warmth begins to build in the area of the pubis, move your left hand in clockwise or counterclockwise circles eighty-one times.

Rub your hands together vigorously again.

Reverse the position of your hands so that your left hand cups the testicles and your right hand is on the pubis. Repeat the circular rubbing in the opposite direction another eighty-one times. Concentrate on what you are doing, and feel the warmth grow. For all Taoist exercises, it is very important — indeed, it is necessary — that you concentrate on the purpose of the physical motions, for doing so will enhance the results. It will unify the body and mind and bring full power to the purpose. Never try to use the mind to force the natural processes by imagining fires growing in the public area, or any other area. This is dangerous.

Second Stage —

Tighten the muscles around the anus and draw them up and in. When done properly, it will feel as if air is being drawn up to your rectum, or as if the entire anal area is being drawn in and upward. Tighten as hard as you can and hold as long as you are able to do so comfortably.

Stop and relax a moment.

Repeat the anal contractions. Do this as many times as you can without feeling discomfort.

As you do the second stage of the exercise, concentrate on feeling a tingling sensation (similar to an electric shock) ascend along the pathway of the Seven Glands. The sensation lasts for fractions of a second and results naturally. Do not try to force this with mental images.

Some teachings suggest that thoughts should be used to help or guide energy flow. Those who make these suggestions misunderstand the nature of energy.

There are six forms of energy: mechanical energy, heat energy, sound energy, radiant energy, atomic energy, and electrical energy. We emit electrical energy. The electrical energy in man differs drastically from that used to run a house, for example. The electrical current in the average house fluctuates at 60 cycles per second; in men, 49,000,000 cycles per second. The latter figure is about half that of light, which travels at 186,000 miles per second. So when a man starts to think or breathe, the electrical energy will have already reached its destination. Our thoughts, breaths, etc. are too slow to guide the flow of electrical energy.

What occurs at the unconscious level was not meant to be subject to the control of the conscious mind. If the conscious mind interfere with something it was not evolved to control—helping or guiding electrical energy through visualization, thoughts, etc.—it can cause a great deal of damage. Its interference with the natural progress of energy can cause schizophrenia, brain damage, and a host of other problems. Taoists call these calamities "Disintegration into Evil."

The Deer Exercise is extremely safe—provided, that it is not supplemented with techniques of other teachings. For show, various incompatible techniques are often thrown together to create spectacular techniques, but the results are often disastrous. Lao-Tse said, "My way is simple and easy." And true Taoist methods *are* simple and easy.

NOTE A: At first you may find that you are able to hold the anal sphincter muscles tight for only a few seconds. Please persist. After several weeks you will be able to hold the muscles tight for quite a while without experiencing weariness or strain.

NOTE B: To determine whether the Deer Exercise is having an effect on the prostate gland, try this test: as you urinate, try to stop the stream of urine entirely through anal muscle contractions. If you are able to do so, then the exercise is effective.

NOTE C: Pressure is being placed on the prostate gland as it is gently massaged by the tightening action of the anal muscles. (The anus can be thought of as a little motor which pumps the prostate gland.) Thus stimulated, the prostate begins to secrete hormones, such as endorphins, etc., to produce a natural high. When the prostate goes into spasms, a small orgasm is experienced. By alternately squeezing and relaxing the anus during the Deer Exercise, a natural high is produced without having to jog ten miles or endure the side-effects of running.

NOTE D: Do this exercise in the morning upon rising and before retiring at night.

VIII

GUARDING THE 'GUARDIAN' —
THE PERIPHERAL PROSTATE MASSAGE

An all-points alert to all those of the male gender who love life: Your prostate needs you!

Fact: Over half of men in western nations over the age of 60 have prostate cancer. Contrast this alarming statistic with the fact that overall cancer rates are much lower in India than in the west; U.S. men get 23 *times* more prostate cancer than men in India. In addition, Americans get between 8 and 14 times the rate of melanoma, 10 to 11 times more colorectal cancer, 9 times more endometrial cancer, 7 to 17 times more lung cancer, 7 to 8 times more bladder cancer, 5 times more breast cancer, and 9 to 12 times more kidney cancer. This is not mere 5, 10, or 20 *percent* more, but 5, 10, or 20 *times* more—or 500%, 1000% and 20,000% more cancer, respectively.

The reason for this apocalyptic cancer tsunami comes down to one simple cause: the highly corrupted Western diet—a disastrous, disease-delivering feast of factory-foods laden with chemicals in the form of pesticides, preservatives, fungicides and color and flavor enhancers— some 1.2 billion pounds of it each year, targeting the nervous system, brain and vital organs, where it wreaks havoc on the cellular metabolism and immune systems.

The Okinawans—among the 3 most disease-free populations on earth thrive on an ancestral diet extremely low in fat, low in protein and low in sugar, as the pie-graph below reveals:

Very simply, then, the Okinawans consume over 90% of their diet as complex carbohydrates, taking 70% in the form of native sweet potatoes, 12% in rice, with another 7% in other grains and 6% in soy products, followed by 4% in various vegetables, 3% fruit and the remainder slender samplings of nuts, other potatoes, seaweed, and barely 1% each in dairy, eggs, fish and meat.

No processed, packaged, industrialized foods; no soft drinks or sweets (consider, a 12-ounce can of Coke contains 9 ½ teaspoons of sugar alone).

When and if Westerners adopt an Okinawan or 7th-Day Adventist plant-based diet, their disease rates plummet to similarly minimal levels—it's that simple.

Beyond the all-powerful realm of a clean, low-fat, low-protein, no-oil, high-carbohydrate diet (contrary to popular mythology, there will be no weight gain—but rather a loss of weight on such a regimen) there are other ways to rescue a failing prostate gland from a cancer diagnosis and the surgeon's knife. The most important of these is the Peripheral Prostate Massage.

People in the virtual era—both men and women—suffer from a great deal of stagnation in the lower pelvis due to lives largely spent sitting for unnaturally prolonged periods of time. While compromising the flexibility of the abdomen, diaphragm and colon, in men, this stagnation impacts the prostate, causing atrophy and hypertrophy due to lack of circulation, oxygen, nutrients and proper detoxification. The prostate surrounds the urethra directly beneath the urinary bladder, and can be felt internally just beyond the ring of the rectal sphincter.

The word 'prostate' derives the from Ancient Greek *prostates*, literally meaning "one who stands before," "protector," or "guardian." The function of the prostate is to secrete a slightly alkaline fluid, milky or white in appearance, that in humans usually constitutes roughly 30% of the volume of the semen along with spermatozoa and seminal vesicle fluid. Semen is made alkaline overall which helps neutralize the acidity of the vaginal tract, prolonging the lifespan of sperm.

A healthy human male prostate is classically said to be slightly larger than a walnut.

Performing a Peripheral Prostate Massage, accessed through the anus, can dramatically restimulate the prostate and restore both flexibility and blood flow, and hence, the health of the organ.

How to Perform the Massage

Place a surgical glove on the active hand.

Start at the '12 o'clock position,' pressing the inserted finger into the center of the surrounding sphincter muscle. While pressing, rub, with a slight in-out motion, for a count of 15 to 20 seconds. Breathe deeply while doing so. This will insure that a maximal level of oxygen in present in the blood that will be flowing through the prostate ring.

Release the pressure, moving to the 3 o'clock position, again pressing inward. As before, massage gently in a small circular motion for a count of 15 to 20 seconds and release.

Repeat this procedure at the 6 and 9 o'clock positions.

The more constricted the anal muscles are, the more discomfort one will feel, ye this should not be taken as reason not to proceed.

As with any massage that loosens up stored stresses, there can be a feeling of tenderness while the body is being reconfigured. Simply take care to avoid any intense pressure or sensations of pain. The goal is to work gently and incrementally enough to feel comfortable in the process.

After completing the first four massages, pause for a while. Then repeat, moving around the circle again, but this time massaging at the points between the initial positions, i.e., between 12 and 3 o'clock, between 3 and 6 o'clock, and so on.

Pause again. Then, perform one more circuit, starting at the 12 o'clock position but this time hitting both the first four positions and the mid-points, i.e., between 12 and 3, then 3, then between 3 and 6. And so on. Massage for just 10 seconds per position on the last round.

Rest and breathe deeply but without effort for a few minutes. The entire massage should take about 15 minutes, which is ample.

Keep in mind that the resting periods between repetitions are vital in order to provide fresh blood and oxygen to nourish and energize the muscles and glands.

You may notice that, upon the third round, everything feels easier. The muscles and the entire body will feel more relaxed, because the anus acts as a reflex point for the entire body.

Following the massage one may feel pleasantly spent, a natural reaction to the release of systemic tension.

Tension keeps you wired. Tension actually stimulates your adrenal system like a drug.

Once the stimulation is removed—and with it, the residual tension that had been stored in the body, one gets a much truer sense of how the body feels, and there is a sense of inner aliveness.

The massage discharges long-stored neurological blockages, and as such utilizes a great deal of energy, so it is best to perform it at a time after which one may deeply rest afterward.

Following the massage, one may experience a period of tenderness for several hours or days—a normal reaction to newly awakened nerves and tissues which may require a period of adjustment.

Toxins have been flushed from the system, and in their transit have sensitized and possibly temporarily inflamed the tissues—a period usually lasting not more than a day or so. Repeated practice will shorten this interval, until it no longer occurs.

One eventually experiences a systemic sense of well-being as a result of regularly performing the massage at 3 to 4 day intervals—enough time to allow for the re-formatting the body requires.

When you reach the point where the Anal Peripheral Prostate Massage feels only good, you can discontinue it until you feel the need for it again.

Once the circulation in this part of the body has been kick-started, it may be maintained not only by periodic prostate massage, but also by taking great care never to sit for more than 20-30 minutes without arising, walking around, doing some squats, hopping on a mini-trampoline for a minute or two, doing some light stretches and bends, deep breathing for 3-5 minutes with a focus upon easily expanding and contracting the diaphragm, or, if one must stay in one's seat due to work requirements, subtly squirming and gyrating in one's chair while contracting and stretching one's legs, feet, buttocks, diaphragm and spine.

IX

THE POTENCY-ENHANCING POWER OF
HOT & COLD HYDROTHERAPY

Dr. Richard Schulze, for many years an alternative healer with a clinic in Santa Monica, California, affirms that of all the many powerful modalities and practices he employed in reversing terminal conditions in over eighty percent of his patients, hydrotherapy was the most powerful and rapid.

He explains that, at one time, hydrotherapy clinics and spas were common on the American landscape, but that today, there are virtually none. In these healing centers, clients were exposed—sometimes for hours—to a vast array of water-based treatment protocols—from steam to total immersion to high-intensity jet-sprays from every direction, which had the effect of stimulating, detoxifying and soothing the body in an exponentially rapid fashion. Indeed, Schulze testifies to the fact that he has seen large tumors reduced by as much as 50% in as little as an hour of alternating hot-cold shower therapy, due to the enhancement of the circulatory and eliminatory systems.

The effect of the hot water is to draw the blood from deep in the body to the surface of the skin, opening and flushing the pores, while the effect of the cold or ice water is to shut down the pores and drive the blood and lymph deep within the vital organs and tissues, in effect, 'rinsing' them of their internal deposits and toxins. When done repeatedly over a sustained period of time, this 'circulatory blitz' has a profound cleansing and healing effects.

A simple way of reaping these benefits is to spend anywhere from 3 gradually up to as much as 30 or more minutes under a shower alternating for 15-30 second intervals between temperatures from as hot to as cold as one can comfortably tolerate, taking care to assure that the entire body is treated—front to back, head to toe.

Finish with a mildly warm flow, taking care to avoid chill afterwards.

The relaxing and invigorating power of this protocol cannot be overestimated. Take care to end with a lukewarm temperature, drying well, and avoiding any chill or cold until the body has a chance to readjust to room temperature.

X

THE SEXUAL REJUVENATION TECHNIQUES OF BERNARR MACFADDEN

Bernarr MacFadden, christened 'The Father of Physical Culture,' was a famous early 20th century American health pioneer who almost died at the age of 7 due to the effects of a botched vaccination, causing him, upon his recovery, to dedicate his life to seeking well-being. He was married for the fourth time when he was 80—to a woman of 44— and lived a long and healthy life, passing away at the ripe old age of 87.

While the style of this excerpt may seem somewhat dated, the insights and techniques are still valid and powerful for contemporary seekers after rejuvenation,

Although Macfadden was not a strict vegetarian, meat was a very minor part of his diet. He preferred carrots to just about any other food. He shunned candies, cakes, pies, and ice cream. He also taught that white bread was one of the worst things a person could eat. He advocated eating in moderation - two meals a day. He said that the 3 meals a day routine killed many people.

He advocated fasting both on a regular basis (He fasted every Monday during his whole life) and when sick. Almost all diseases could be cured by the correct fasting regimen.

He was strongly in favor of drinking whole milk. He even prescribed a milk diet for some ailments. He opposed pasteurization and homogenization of milk.

He was against the use of tobacco, alcohol, and drugs, even drugs prescribed by doctors. He said that most doctors are just "pill pushers" who treat symptoms. To treat a disease, the cause needed to be removed. He opposed vaccinations. (As a child, he had almost died from a poorly executed vaccination.)

He told people that they need to exercise regularly. His favorite form of exercise was walking. Besides walking several miles each day, he also organized walks that were hundreds of miles long. His method of walking was brisk, to say the least. He also prescribed calisthenics and training with light weights.

He taught that hair growth can be stimulated and that 20-20 eyesight could be restored. He told people that they should never wear eyeglasses, but do exercises to correct their vision. For toothache he prescribed chewing on pieces of wood!

He opposed women wearing corsets or any kind of restrictive clothing. He advocated wearing loose fitting clothes. He believed that the best shoes had no heels and were open like sandals. He went barefoot whenever he could, because he said that the energy of the earth came up through his feet that way.

He taught that sex and the sex drive were good and natural and that prudery and ignorance fostered all kinds of social ills.

He believed in sleeping on a firm surface. He mostly slept on the floor all during his life. He believed in having fresh air in a well ventilated room while a person is sleeping. Sleeping outdoors during warm weather was best.

He spoke out against the stranglehold that organized medicine had on health care in America. He spoke in favor of licensing drugless practitioners and midwives, naturopaths, homeopaths, and chiropractors. He advocated natural childbirth and that mothers nurse their babies.

He taught that air baths and exposure to sunlight were good and healthful. He believed that a cold plunge built strength and endurance. He is supposed to have been the founder of the Polar Bear clubs.

He believed that energy, determination, courage, and an iron will were vital to lasting health. He believed that physical exercise stimulated the brain to think better.

He stated that by his methods all diseases could be cured including: all forms of cancer, tuberculosis, diabetes, and venereal diseases.

He was the first to propose that the President should have a National Secretary of Health on his cabinet.

The excerpt that follows is from his book, *Manhood and Marriage*.

"I HAVE in the past devoted a great deal of attention to what I consider the great importance of exercise in the building of virility. Whenever you add to your vitality you in-crease your nervous energy and in consequence add to the virile powers of the body. The more perfect you make yourself as a man, the more complete you will become in every way and the more you will have to perpetuate. If you are so fragile and defective that you are not worth perpetuating, then as a natural consequence you lose, or never develop, the virile powers of perfect man-hood.

"Physical activity means exercise for the internal organs as well as for the muscles, and therefore every cell in the body partakes of the benefit. Through the influence on the circulation, exercise has the effect of flushing all parts of, the body with fresh, pure, oxygenated blood and thus has an internal cleansing effect. Dead cells and waste matter are carried away, new building material is supplied, oxygen is brought to every tissue and cell in the most remote extremities, and accordingly every tissue and every cell is filled with life and energy.

"Muscular stagnation means a wasting away of the muscles themselves, but it also means much more than this. It means sluggish circulation and a poorer quality of blood. It means inactivity and imperfect functioning of the various vital organs. It means also a lessening of virility. No man can be sexually normal unless he is physically vigorous and fully alive in every respect. The physical weakling either is or shortly becomes a sexual weakling, for impotence tends to follow directly upon long-continued muscular inactivity. The man who so degenerates in respect to his all-round physical vigor that he is only a mockery of a man is no longer fit and worthy to perpetuate his kind, and the functional channel through which propagation is accomplished deteriorates accordingly.

"Therefore, in order to regain your lost manhood, if you have been weakened in this respect, make up your mind to adopt a suitable course of physical training with a view to making a real man of yourself from a muscular or athletic standpoint. You may rest assured that by the time you have reached the general physical condition and vigor of an athlete you will have little to complain of in respect to your sexual condition.

"Carrying this idea of exercise as a body and vitality builder to its logical conclusion with reference to this subject, I have recently carried out some studies and experiments which have resulted in some remarkable discoveries in connection with the development of unusual virility. As I have often explained, virility depends to a large extent upon nervous energy, the harmonious working of the nervous powers of the body. The sexual system and the general physical organism act and react upon each other in accordance with the condition of each. For instance, if you are suffering from spermatorrhea, or from any losses due to the weakness of the muscles of the glands that are intended to retain the life-giving fluids of the body, such losses will naturally affect the general physical organism quite materially. Every drop of these vital fluids is weighted with a tremendous amount of energy, and their loss represents so much wasted force.

"The problem is to restore the vigorous muscular tone of this organ and increase the strength of the entire generative system, including the ejaculatory ducts, the seminal vesicles and the posterior urethra. Remember also that seminal losses, particularly in spermatorrhea, and prostatorrhea as well, result from a weakened condition of these parts. The loss of prostate fluid is due entirely to a relaxed and dilated condition of the prostatic ducts. It is essential that these should be contracted, and that all the tissues, muscles and nerves involved should be toned up. Local cold-water treatment, exercises that promote the circulation, and all helpful influences generally, will tend to restore these tissues to a normal condition. But exercise of these parts themselves will directly strengthen them, and that is the purpose of the new method of which I am speaking.

"The idea occurred to me that if means could be found actually to exercise the muscular tissue of the prostate gland, great advantages would be se-cured thereby. The location of the prostate gland itself indicates what, to my mind, is a wise provision on the part of the Creator for the purpose of maintaining the functional vigor of this very important organ. It is well known that if a muscle lies inactive for an indefinite time it becomes soft and flaccid or, even, in some cases, entirely loses its power. Now, the peculiar location of the prostate gland—surrounding the urethra at the neck of the bladder—insures that it is exercised every day, to a certain extent in connection with the passage of the urine. That this remarkable provision of nature is designed to maintain virility in spite of continence continued over a very prolonged period seems very clear. The means of further exercising this gland was easily learned.

"You have probably noticed that you have some degree of control over these parts, for probably every one immediately at the end of the act of urinating tries to force out of the urethral canal the few remaining drops by means of a muscular contraction at the neck of the bladder and in the region of the perineum generally. The muscles concerned you can learn to contract voluntarily, and as you practice the exercise you will find that you do it better and better.

"There is little need for going into details about the value of exercises of this sort. They have been found in practice to be unusually helpful, and their value will be self-evident to anyone who cares to give the idea a brief trial. I am therefore offering a series of what might be termed internal tensing movements, or "Prostate Gland Tensing Movements," the object of which is the acceleration of the circulation and the improvement of the tissues directly affecting sexuality.

"Also, while searching for more definite knowledge on this most important subject, I noted the location of the nerves of the spine that radiate to the sexual organs. It seemed conclusive to me that by exercising this particular part of the spine in a vigorous manner, these nerves would be stimulated to function more vigorously and perfectly, thus increasing virility and general stamina. In what is known as the upper lumbar region of the spine, at about "the small" of the back, are located the vertebrae from which issue the spinal nerves that control and supply the energy for the entire sexual system. I am, accordingly, including in this list of exercises some very effective movements for strengthening and stimulating this particular part of the back. They have been named "Lower Spinal Tensing Movements."

"Phrenologists have maintained that the seat of the affections, or the emotions influenced by the sexual system, is located at the lower back part of the brain. Now, there is no method of directly exercising the brain in the manner that we exercise a muscle, but the idea occurred to me that by strengthening the muscles at the base of the skull, that is, those located at the back of the neck, one would, to a certain extent, influence the sexual function. I am therefore presenting a method of exercising these muscles under the head of "Upper Spinal Tensing Movements." In addition I am suggesting some entirely new ideas for exercising the muscular tissue adjacent to the sexual system which will undoubtedly have a very decided effect if done regularly. Please note, however, that if there is any doubt as to the condition of the heart, kidneys and blood pressure an examination by a dependable physician in sympathy with these theories is suggested.

PROSTATE GLAND TENSING MOVEMENTS

"The best way to acquire the ability to tense the muscles of the prostate gland is to stop the passage of the urine frequently when evacuating the bladder. The muscles concerned are those used to check or control the flow of the urine, and after you have acquired the ability to tense these muscles at will, it will be advisable each time immediately after passing water to tense them from five to ten times, according to your inclination. Don't overdo the exercise. An error of this sort might result in an enlarged prostate, and this is far from pleasant. There are other internal muscles in this region which should also be included in these contractions, particularly those about the rectum and anus. I do not refer here to those voluntary muscles in the abdomen with which one sometimes assists in the movement of the bowels, but rather to those with which one resists the impulse to move the bowels. Get control of these and learn to contract or tense them vigorously along with the muscles of the prostate gland and surrounding parts.

"A few contractions of these tissues will not count for much, but if you make the movements frequently it will mean a great improvement in the course of a little time. You can practice them when sitting at a desk, and you will perhaps find that you can contract the muscles more vigorously if you press the knees together at the same time, or cross the legs. You might make it a rule to do this not only after urinating, but also ten or twenty times morning, noon and night, and perhaps at other times during the day.

"It is a good plan also, at frequent intervals when urinating, to use considerable effort with a view to forcing out the urine as fast as possible. This of course to a certain extent exercises all these muscles, in addition to the muscular tissues of the bladder and abdomen generally. I consider this plan invaluable in the treatment of stricture, since forcing the stream in this manner is naturally inclined to enlarge the opening and assist in remedying any obstruction of the passage.

LOWER SPINAL TENSING MOVEMENTS

"To acquire the ability to tense the muscles of the lower spine place the end of one finger upon the spinous process or bony structure of the spine in the small of the back, and the other fingers on the muscles on each side. Then,

104

through the mere effort of your will, tense the muscles in this region vigorously. You may find this difficult at first, but if you are fairly muscular, you will soon secure full control of these muscles. You should practice these tensing movements or contractions of the muscles until tired two or three times a day, or whenever you find it convenient. The exercise can be taken when slightly bent forward, while standing erect, or while lying down. If you practice them with sufficient regularity you will actually be amazed at the change in the character of the muscular tissue in the small of the back. Furthermore, you will notice a tendency to stand erect, and an absence of that weakness of the spine which is such a tremendous handicap to those suffering from sexual weakness of any sort. Later in this chapter I shall refer to some supplementary exercises for the spine, for those who have time, but I would particularly urge careful attention to these spinal tensing movements in all cases. Practice them faithfully and persistently if you wish good results.

UPPER SPINAL TENSING MOVEMENTS

"Control of the upper spinal muscles may be acquired in the same manner as in the case of the lower ones. Place the fingers on the back of the neck just below the base of the skull, and endeavor, through an effort of the will, to tense the muscles, avoiding as far as possible any contraction of the muscles in the front of the neck. Give your entire attention to the muscles on the back of the neck. "Concentrate" your thoughts there. If the muscles are well developed, little effort will be required to obtain full control of them; other-wise it may take some time. When you are able to tense them at will, you will not need to depend upon placing your hand thereon. You can tell by the feeling of the muscles themselves that they are being properly tensed.

"The exercise can be taken while sitting, standing or reclining, though as a rule control is more easily obtained in the beginning in a standing position. It may be repeated two or three times a day, or whenever convenient, provided that your efforts are not continued beyond ordinary, fatigue at any time.

"The exercising of the spinal muscles has a tendency to strengthen and stimulate the spine generally, and this also must react favorably upon the sexual system. At the same time the use of these muscles will tend to make you sit and stand more erect, giving you a better and more manly appearance, and all this has a mental effect outside of its physiological influence.

"In addition to these special exercises, I would par-ticularly suggest the following movements which are entirely new and which can be strongly recommended for the building of virility. Each one of these movements may be taken at almost any time of the day when convenient, and may be continued until a feeling of fatigue is induced.

BEARING-DOWN EXERCISE

"This movement has a peculiarly beneficial effect upon the internal organs located in the lower part of the abdominal region. It consists in bearing down slightly just as one would when endeavoring to move the bowels. Care should of course be taken when beginning this exercise to avoid strain of any kind, especially in the case of one suffering from spermatorrhea or from rupture. In fact, when these two complaints are present it might be well to avoid the exercise altogether, or at least to do it very lightly and infrequently. What is termed "straining at stool" is supposed to be injurious when there is the slightest tendency toward spermatorrhea, but in the exercise as above described there need be no strain, merely pressure that can be regulated in such a manner as to avoid strain of any sort. Continue the movement each time until a slight feeling of fatigue is noticed.

DRAWING IN THE ABDOMEN

"This exercise is of special value in increasing abdominal strength, and consists simply in the drawing in of the lower abdominal region to the fullest extent of your capacity. If one is not fairly well developed in this region the exercise may be difficult at first, but by practice you will soon be able to obtain full control over these muscles. Draw the abdomen in as far as you possibly can, relax, and then repeat the exercise, continuing until a sense of fatigue is noticed.

HIP TENSING EXERCISE

"The easiest way to learn this exercise is to attempt it when standing erect. Tense the muscles of the extreme upper legs and of the buttocks, placing the hands on the muscles so that you may be able to determine whether or not you are properly performing the exercise. When correctly executed, you will feel the muscles harden under your touch each time you tense them. The circulation of the blood through the hips and upper legs is very greatly accelerated by this movement, and the improvement in the quality of the tissues adjacent to the sexual parts un-doubtedly has an influence of special value.

SPINE STRETCHING EXERCISE

"The object of this exercise is to stretch and tense the spine throughout its entire length, thus arousing to greater activity practically every organ of the body, and one of its ad-vantages is that it can be taken anywhere, whether sitting, standing or walking. Simply endeavor to bring the head upward and backward as far as you can, stretching the spine and flexing its muscles throughout its every part as vigorously as you possibly can. Re-lax and repeat the exercise until a feeling of fatigue is induced.

"I regard the above exercise as being of unusual importance in virility building, and have there-fore called special attention to them, but, of course, additional exercises will help. The movements referred to in the few pages following may be regarded as supplementary. If you have time enough, you can map out an exclusive course of training. But if your strength is limited in the beginning, or if you have very little time, you will get most benefit from the special exercises outlined above.

"Now taking up ordinary exercises for the external muscles, I may say that there are two or even three types which should receive careful attention: first, special movements which affect the sexual region in a stimulating manner; second, general exercises for all around bodily vigor; and third, additional spinal exercises for stimulating the nervous system and thus reacting upon the generative system.

"The first type of exercises, consisting of special movements of a stimulating nature, are particularly valuable in the treatment of varicocele, and are useful also in the case of impotence or "lost manhood." In the ease of those suffering from masturbation, night losses, spermatorrhea or prematurity, in whom there is already over stimulation of the sex organs they are of value but not so desirable as in the former conditions. These cases especially require the general exercises for all-round vigor. The exercises for the spine are valuable in every instance.

"The special stimulating exercises of most value for local strengthening of the sex organs, are those which bring into action the muscles of the adjacent parts of the body, notably the abdomen, the hips and the upper thighs, especially the adductor muscles of the thighs. Such exercises not only strengthen the particular muscles concerned, but they also strengthen, and increase the circulation in all the adjacent organs and tissues.

"These special exercises will naturally consist of such movements as the following: Lying on. the back, raise the hips off the floor as high as posible. Lying on the stomach, raise legs and shoulders high from the floor, with hands behind the back. Lying on the back, flex the knees tightly against the abdomen, either one at a time, or both together. Lying on the back, raise the legs to perpendicular position. Lying on the back, raise one leg at a time to the perpendicular, then endeavor to swing it inward across the body. Lying on the right side, place the weight of the lower body on the left or upper foot, and try to raise the hips slightly. Similar movement on left side. Lying on the back, with feet held firm, rise to sitting position. Lying on the side, swing the upper, leg upward as high as possible.

Lying face downward, raise one leg at a time up-ward and backward as high as possible. Lying on the back, swing the right leg over the left and stretch it as far across to the left as you can. Same with left leg to the right side. Lying on the back, with knees doubled against chest, kick upward alternately with each leg. Better yet if a heavy pillow is placed under the hips to elevate them.

"Any other exercise that you may devise that affects the same general region of the body may be used. Any movements of the legs that involve the "scissors" action, or which approach the acrobatic feat known as the "split," will more or less affect this region. Swimming is a capital exercise because the action of the legs, whether it be in the scissors or frog kick, is exactly suited to the requirements under consideration, and in fact swimming is of unusual value in building general vitality as well as virility. Fast running is also effective in the same way, but it is such a violent exercise for a debilitated man that he must be very careful in the beginning not to exhaust himself. High kicking is another exercise which may be commended, like running, after one has gained a material degree of strength. High kicking would be suggested in a case of varicocele, if there is not too much tenderness and pain.

"In a case of varicocele or much congestion of the prostate gland, it might be advantageous to relieve the blood pressure in this region, at least so far as the veins are concerned, by assuming an upside-down position for two or three minutes at a time, and by executing some special exercises in that position. An elevated position of the hips, secured through the use of pillows, or lying on an inclined plane, head downward, would be satisfactory; or, what would be a little more strenuous .but also more effective, you could assume a position balanced on the shoulders and back of the head. Lying first on the back, raise the legs, extending them upward and raising the hips and back until you can rest the elbows on the floor and support the small of the back at each side with your hands, practically standing on the back of your shoulders. In this position you can spread the legs apart and bring them together again, execute a scissors movement, double the legs and then kick them up, and perform other movements which you may be able to work out for yourself. This position and these exercises will tend to get the stagnant blood out of the congested parts. Remember that in the upright position of the body peculiar to the human race there is a considerable column of blood in the large veins which must be forced upward to the heart. The large abdominal veins are sometimes greatly distended, with much pressure. The above position will relieve this and favor the movement of the blood in the smaller congested veins. I would particularly recommend this treatment when a case of varicocele is accompanied by much pain.

"Usually if the heart and other organs are healthy and in tone it will be desirable to combine the special exercises which I have described with general body-building movements. For in all cases one must build all-round bodily vigor. It would be best to use the general and spinal exercises first each morning, then after the general circulation has been aroused, to take the special exercises for the purpose of concentrating the circulation, to some extent, in the region of the genital organs. Finally take a friction rub and a cold sitz-bath. Altogether, this might take up thirty or forty minutes, perhaps less. Don't be too strenuous at first, for all these exercises are very effective. Don't continue to the point of exhaustion. Feel your way carefully in the matter of exercise, and gradually become more energetic. As I have said, when the sex organs are already over-stimulated, as in masturbation, seminal losses and prematurity, it will be just as well to avoid the special exercises, and confine yourself to the spinal movements and those for general body building.

"A form of exercise or massage which will be found stimulating in cases of complete impotence, is percussion of the abdomen. This is particularly effective in relieving constipation, and will also help a weak bladder and influence the prostate gland. It consists in a rapid tapping or pounding of the abdomen with the tips of the fingers, the sides of the hands, or the fists, according to how strong you may be and how vigorous you desire to make the treatment. But it should not be attempted when there is inflammation or congestion of any of the parts, or if one suffers from seminal losses.

"We now come to the subject of general exercises for building all-round bodily vigor which are necessary in every case, of whatsoever kind. It is not my purpose to insist upon any particular kind of movements for this purpose, because you may choose to vary your exercise for the sake of interest. The kind of general exercise does not matter so much as the fact that you actually get it, and thus build general strength. Build up every part of the body as thoroughly as possible.

"In order that you may not overlook the importance of this, let me emphasize again with all possible force, the intimate relation between general physical weakness and sexual debility. The muscular weakling positively cannot expect to become sexually vigorous until he builds up a robust condition of body.

"I am convinced, in fact, that it is practically impossible for one to continue to suffer from a disorder like varicocele, prostatic congestion, or congestion of any other part of the body, if he daily engages in a sufficient amount of athletic exercise to keep the blood circulating vigorously for any length of time. Without any special treatment the improvement in the general circulation would inevitably restore a normal circulation and a healthy condition in the diseased parts. In other words, the athletic man may not only endure more abuse, but he can the more readily overcome the results of any abuse which he may have suffered. I can promise that long-continued and active exercise like distance running, tennis, handball, clog dancing, rope skip-ping, or very fast walking, by bringing about and maintaining for two or three hours at a time an unusually active circulation throughout every minute tissue of the body, would very quickly dispose of any case of varicocele, or congestion of the urethra, prostate or other parts. If you can take daily exercise of this kind, almost athletic in character, in connection with any special or development exercise needed, and thereby influence the general circulation in this way for two or three hours at a time, you will find that it will exert a powerful curative influence.

"I realize that the sexually weak man is usually too debilitated at first to follow out any such vigorous program. He should not attempt it in the beginning. But it represents the ideal toward which he should work. He should gradually build himself up until he has attained this athletic quality and his body is a picture of normal muscular development. This is possible at any age. Don't think that you have to be under twenty or any other age to develop yourself.

"Above everything I recommend walking as a constitutional tonic and general exercise for building endurance and vital stamina. If you are not strong, start in with moderate walks, continuing only until slightly fatigued. Don't half-kill yourself. Each day slightly increase the distance until you are able to cover ten or fifteen miles without special inconvenience. You should reach that condition in three months in most cases, perhaps sooner, and when you can walk ten miles without being tired, you will be making fine progress. Don't poke along in a lazy manner. Step out briskly, so as to induce deep breathing and even perspiration. That's the kind of walk that will build vitality.

"Do not forget what I have said about the tonic effect of outdoor life of any kind. Try to live in the open for a time, and as you get stronger indulge in as many open-air pastimes as you can. Splitting wood I consider an ideal strength-building exercise, but don't exhaust yourself in the beginning. Pitching hay is another superb exercise, and farm work in general can be recommended. Climbing trees, if you are in the country, is one of the most pleasant and most satisfactory exercises that I can suggest. Swimming I have already mentioned. But as you become sufficiently vigorous I would by all means recommend such energetic games as handball, tennis, baseball, football, hockey, boxing, and wrestling. Horseback riding is of doubtful value in cases in which there is congestion or irritability of the prostate gland, or possibly aggravated varicocele. Remember that open air life builds nerve

strength, as well as muscular vigor, and that you particularly need to build up the nervous forces of the body.

"The spinal exercises are of exceptional importance as a
means of invigorating the central nervous system. To the
spinal tensing movements which I have specially advised,
you may add other exercises which affect the muscles and
ligaments of the back, and especially those which tend to
stretch the back bone. In fact, all body stretching and
trunk-bending exercises may be considered as suitable for
the spine, but for the present purpose one should give
particular attention to movements that affect the small of
the back.

> While hanging by the hands from some support,
> preferably against the side of a high fence, wall or
> door, bend or raise the legs far backward from the
> hips. This affects the lower spine.

> Also, for the same purpose, lying face downward,
> and holding the shoulders down by taking hold of
> something, raise the legs as high as you can from the
> hips. Lying face down, with legs held down, raise
> head, shoulders and chest as high as you can.

> Standing with hands on hips, feet apart, bend far
> backward and for-ward; also twist, from the waist,
> far to each side. Then circle the body around, rotating
> from the hips, first in one direction, then in the other.

> While stretching the back, with arms high above the
> head, bend far to each side.

All of these movements will directly affect the part of the spine that you desire to influence for this purpose, though of course other exercises for the upper spine, including neck bending and stretching, will naturally help, through their general stimulating effect upon the entire nervous system. I may say that I have given considerable attention to spinal exercises in my book, *Vitality Supreme*, but those I have mentioned here will cover your needs for the purpose under consideration. Perform each movement only a few times, for they are extremely energizing and effective, but don't be lazy in their execution.

"The time to take your exercise will depend somewhat upon your work. It may sometimes be necessary to take it in the evening. I would lay down no rules, except that it is not best to exercise just before going to bed when you find it too stimulating. A good plan in most cases is to do the formal exercises in the morning, first general development movements, then spinal exercises, then the special movements, following them by a quick friction rub and a cold sitz-bath. If the cold sitz is not suited to your case, take a cold sponge bath instead. Take your walk or other outdoor exercise later in the day, preferably late in the afternoon, but in the evening if your work makes this necessary.

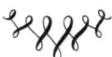

Recommended Further Reading

Daniel P. Reid: The Tao of Health, Sex & Longevity;
Touchstone, 1989

Mantak Chia: Taoist Secrets of Love: Cultivating Male
Sexual Energy; Aurora Press 1984

Healing Love Through the Tao; Destiny Books, 2005

Paavo Airola: Sex and Nutrition, Mass Market Paperback
1975

JOSEPH ANDREW MARCELLO

Joseph Andrew Marcello is an award-winning composer and author, with books on subjects as varied as Qigong healing (*Life More Abundant: the Science of Zhineng Qigong*, Infinity Publishing) and film music (*The Wolf Man*, MagicImage Books); mysticism (*Living Vision—The Spiritual Secrets of Neville Lancelot Goddard*, CreateSpace/Amazon) . His most recent work is *The Healing Power of Pyramids*, (Amazon CreateSpace), an exploration of the beneficial energies of sacred geometries.

A lifelong composer, he is the recipient of the Delius Award for Composers for his virtuosic piano suite, *Dances of the Night*, and has created works in all genres—from opera to musicals, from choral to orchestral to chamber music. His forthcoming CD album is entitled *Glory— Spirituals for Our Time*.

He dwells on a pine-clad hilltop in Western Massachusetts with his 13 cockatiels, where he writes, composes and indulges his passions for long-distance swimming and hugging trees. He may be reached by email at: JosephMarcello@verizon.net

EMILE RAUX

Alas, repeated research has yielded no information on this mysterious author—to whom the contemporary western world owes a great debt of gratitude, nonetheless.